Astrogliosis and Channel Function

John V. Zimmerman

Astrogliosis is a hallmark of central nervous system (CNS) neuroinflammatory disorders such as multiple sclerosis (MS). Astrocytes can play both beneficial and detrimental roles in response to neuroinflammation, thus a detailed understanding of the underlying molecular mechanisms governing astrogliosis might facilitate the development of therapeutic targets. While astrocytes do not express voltage-gated sodium channel (VGSC) Nav1.5 in nonpathological human brain, they exhibit robust upregulation of Navi .5 within acute and chronic MS lesions. We investigated the contribution of voltage-gated sodium channels to astrogliosis in an *in vitro* model of mechanical injury to astrocytes. Previous studies have shown that a scratch injury to astrocytes invokes dual mechanisms of migration and proliferation in these cells. Our results demonstrate that wound closure after mechanical injury, involving both migration and proliferation, is attenuated by pharmacological treatment with tetrodotoxin (TTX) and KB-R7943, at a dose that blocks reverse mode of the Na^+/Ca^{2+} exchanger (NCX), and by knockdown of Navi .5 mRNA. We also show that astrocytes display a robust $[Ca^{2+}]_i$ transient after mechanical injury and demonstrate that this $[Ca^{2+}]_i$ response is also attenuated by TTX, KB-R7943, and Navi .5 mRNA knockdown. This study provides support for a contribution of VGSCs in the pathway leading to astrogliosis.

We present here evidence supporting a contribution of sodium channel Nav1.5 to astrogliosis in an *in vitro* model of glial mechanical injury. We further implicate fluctuations in $[Ca^{2+}]_i$ due to reverse operation of NCX, triggered by VGSC activity, as a mechanism by which Nav1.5 contributes to the response of astrocytes to mechanical injury. Our results establish a link between the activity of VGSCs and astrogliosis by way of alterations in $[Ca^{2+}]_i$. Here we show, in an *in vitro* model of mechanical injury to astrocytes, that voltage-gated sodium channel (VGSC) Nav1.5, traditionally viewed as a cardiac sodium channel, contributes to the astrocytic response to the insult via triggering reverse mode of the Na^+/Ca^{2+} exchanger (NCX).

We then investigated the temporal dynamics of astrocytic Nav1.5 channel expression in response to neuroinflammatory pathologies. We examined astrocytes from mice with monophasic and chronic-relapsing experimental autoimmune encephalomyelitis (EAE) by immunohistochemistry to determine whether Nav1.5 is expressed in these cells, and whether the expression correlates with severity of disease and/or phases of relapse and remission. Our results demonstrate that Nav1.5 is upregulated in astrocytes *in situ* in a temporal manner that correlates with disease severity in both monophasic and chronic-relapsing EAE. Furthermore, in chronic-relapsing EAE, Nav1.5 expression is upregulated during relapses and subsequently attenuated during periods of remission. These observations are consistent with the suggestion that Nav1.5 can play a role in the response of astrocytes to inflammatory pathologies in the

CNS and suggest Nav1.5 may be a potential therapeutic target to modulate reactive astrogliosis *in vivo*.

Finally, we investigated whether Nav1.5 expression in astrocytes plays a role in the pathogenesis of EAE. We created a conditional knockout of Nav1.5 in astrocytes and determined whether this affects the clinical course of EAE, focal macrophage and T cell infiltration, and diffuse activation of astrocytes. We show that deletion of Nav1.5 from astrocytes leads to significantly worsened clinical outcomes in EAE, with increased inflammatory infiltrate in both early and late stages of disease, unexpectedly, in a sex-specific manner. Removal of Nav1.5 in astrocytes leads to increased inflammation in female mice with EAE, including increased astroglial response and infiltration of T cells and phagocytic monocytes. These cellular changes are consistent with more severe EAE clinical scores. Additionally, we found evidence suggesting possible dysregulation of the immune response – particularly regarding infiltrating macrophages and activated microglia – in female Nav1.5 KO mice compared to WT littermate controls. Together, our results show that deletion of Nav1.5 from astrocytes leads to significantly worsened clinical outcomes in EAE, with increased inflammatory infiltrate in both early and late stages of disease, in a sex-specific manner.

TABLE OF CONTENTS

<u>CHAPTER 1</u>: Introduction

1.2.1 Multiple sclerosis

1.2.2 Experimental autoimmune encephalomyelitis

1.2.3 Estrogens and neuroprotection

1.3.1 Noncanonical expression and functions

1.3.2 Glial expression of sodium channels

1.3.3 Functional role of sodium channels in glia

<u>CHAPTER 2</u>: Functional role of Nav1.5 in astrogliosis in vitro

2.3.1 Astrocytes express Nav1.5 and NCX1

2.3.2 TTX and KB-R7943 inhibit astroglial response to injury

2.3.3 Nav1.5 knockdown inhibits astrocyte response to injury

<u>CHAPTER 3</u>: Dynamics of Nav1.5 expression in astrocytes in mouse models of multiple sclerosis

LIST OF TABLES AND FIGURES

ACM	astrocyte-conditioned medium
AP-1	activator protein 1
ATP	adenosine triphosphate
AUC	area under the curve
BBB	blood-brain barrier
BrdU	bromodeoxyuridine
$[Ca^{2+}]_i$	intracellular calcium
CCL2	chemokine (C-C motif) ligand 2
CD3	cluster of differentiation 3
CD11b	cluster of differentiation 11b
CD45	cluster of differentiation 45
cDNA	complementary deoxyribonucleic acid
CFA	complete Freud's adjuvant
CNS	central nervous system
CR EAE	chronic-relapsing experimental autoimmune encephalomyelitis
CTL	control
EAE	experimental autoimmune encephalomyelitis
ECM	extracellular matrix
EDSS	expanded disability status scale
ERK	extracellular signal-related kinase
ES cells	embryonic stem cells
GABA	gamma-Aminobutyric acid
GAPDH	glyceraldehyde 3-phosphate dehydrogenase
GFAP	glial fibrillary acidic protein
GTP	guanosine triphosphate
Iba1	ionized calcium-binding adapter molecule 1
i.p.	intraperitoneal
IL	interleukin
KB-R7943	2-[2-[4-(4-Nitrobenzyloxy)phenyl]ethyl] isothiourea mesylate

KO	knockout
LPS	lipopolysaccharide
MAPK	mitogen-activated protein kinase
MCP-1	monocyte chemoattractant protein 1
mGFAP	mouse glial fibrillary acidic protein
MOG	myelin oligodendrocyte glycoprotein
MRI	magnetic resonance imaging
mRNA	messenger ribonucleic acid
MS	multiple sclerosis
$[Na^+]_i$	intracellular sodium
NAWM	normal-appearing white matter
NCX	sodium-calcium exchanger
neo	neomycin
NG2	neural/glial antigen 2
NOS	nitric oxide synthase
n.s.	not significant
NT siRNA	non-targeting silencing ribonucleic acid
OGB	Oregon-Green 488 BAPTA-AM
OX-42	see CD11b
PBS	phosphate-buffered saline
PCR	polymerase chain reaction
PFA	paraformaldehyde
Phen	phenytoin
PP-MS	primary progressive multiple sclerosis
PMA	phorbol-12-myristate-13-acetate
PTx	Pertussis toxin
RA	rheumatoid arthritis
Rac1	Ras-related C3 botulinum toxin substrate 1
RCA	Ricinus communis agglutinin I
RGB	red green blue
RNA	ribonucleic acid

RNFL	retinal nerve fiber layer
ROI	region of interest
ROS	reactive oxygen species
RR-MS	relapsing-remitting multiple sclerosis
RT-PCR	real-time polymerase chain reaction
SBS	standard bath solution
SCI	spinal cord injury
SEM	standard error of the mean
siRNA	silencing ribonucleic acid
SLE	systemic lupus erythematosus
SP-MS	secondary progressive multiple sclerosis
STAT3	signal transducer and activator of transcription 3
STX	saxitoxin
TB	tuberculosis
TBI	traumatic brain injury
TGF-α	transforming growth factor alpha
TTX	tetrodotoxin
TTX-R	tetrodotoxin-resistant
TTX-S	tetrodotoxin-sensitive
VGSC	voltage-gated sodium channel
WT	wild-type

This work would not have been possible without the guidance and unwavering support of my mentor, Stephen Waxman, who is the ultimate example of a physician-scientist. I would like to thank him for finding a place for me in his lab as a medical student, encouraging me to join the Yale MSTP, and for four productive years as his PhD student. He has shown me how indispensable basic research is to the practice of clinical medicine, a lesson I will take throughout my career. He has also been an inspiring example of how to run a large, successful laboratory and a clinical department at a major academic center. He has deeply supported me on both a professional and a personal level, and I am very grateful.

I would like to thank Joel Black, who has been a close mentor and taught me everything from immunocytochemistry to how to write a proper research article. He guided me daily and I appreciate his calm attitude toward the many difficulties that arise in research. Even after moving across the world, he continued to support me to the completion of my PhD, for which I am appreciative.

I would also like to thank my thesis committee for their encouragement, guidance, and support. I am grateful for their ability and willingness to draw out my strengths and constructively identify my weaknesses. Will Cafferty, my committee chair, has been a wonderful mentor and someone I've sought advice from since taking his class several years ago. He willingly opened his lab, teaching me many aspects of spinal cord injury science, spent many hours reading with me for my qualifying exam, and always made himself available to discuss my research. Marina Picciotto interviewed me for the MSTP program 5 years ago and has enthusiastically supported my progress since. She chaired my qualifying committee and her feedback on my thesis research has significantly improved the work. Charlie Greer has been crucial to my continued progress and has ensured that things have proceeded smoothly. I would also like to thank the other members of my qualifying committee for dedicating their time and energy: Jeff Kocsis, Jaime Grutzendler, and Marc Freeman.

I would like to express my gratitude to the faculty and staff of the MD/PhD program. Jim Jamieson was the first person I spoke with about applying to the program, and he has been supportive and encouraging since that initial conversation as a first-year medical student. Barbara Kazmierczak has done a wonderful job continuing that support, and I am grateful for the candid talks we have had about research and career paths. I would also like to thank Cheryl DeFilippo, Sue Sansone, Fred Gorelick, and Tamar Taddei for their many forms of encouragement over the years.

I would like to thank other members of the Waxman lab for their teaching and friendship. Sulayman Dib-Hajj has always been freely giving of his scientific knowledge and advice. Much of this work would not have been possible without assistance from Shujun Liu – my "lab mom" – who has made sure things have gone smoothly since I joined lab. She has been indispensable to many aspects of my dissertation work, and I am grateful for her teaching. Pam Zwinger has played an integral role in the animal work presented here and I admire her dedication and patience. Omar Samad was instrumental to many of the *in vitro* experiments and to the generation of the mouse colony. Palak Shah and Fadia Dib-Hajj played major roles in much of the molecular work, and Mark Estacion assisted with imaging of all kinds. I am also grateful for the friendship and support of many other former and current members of the lab: Betsy Schulman, Lakshmi Bangalore, Talia Adi, Liz Akin, Andrew Tan, Anna-Karin Persson, Philip Effraim, Jianying Huang, Yang Yang, Chongyang Han, Lubin Chen, Maggie Mis, Peng Zhao, Daria Sizova, Myriam Hill, Brian Tanaka, Bhagi Dash, and Curtis Benson. I will miss you all and always think fondly on my time in the lab.

I owe much of my success to my parents, Bob and Jean Ann West. They provided a wonderful and supportive environment growing up and have always encouraged me to be my best self. Their unwavering love and endless support have been essential to where I am today, and words cannot express my gratitude. Finally, I would like to thank my husband, Joey, for being my rock through this degree (and everything else). He has literally been by my side since the week I started in lab and has been patient, kind, and eternally optimistic as I tackled the various challenges presented over the last several years. I'm not quite sure how I got so lucky, but I am very grateful. Finally, I'd like to dedicate this dissertation to my daughter, Amalia, with whom I was 6 months pregnant when I defended this work. She has changed everything for the better.

<u>CHAPTER 1</u>: INTRODUCTION

This chapter contains a modified version of material that appeared in the author's publication: Pappalardo LW, Black JA, Waxman SG (2016). Sodium channels in astroglia and microglia. Glia 64:1628-1645.

1.1   ASTROGLIOSIS

Astrocytes are the most abundant cell population in the human central nervous system (CNS) and are crucial for many functions in the healthy CNS. Astrocytes are a heterogeneous population, and depending on location in the CNS, their roles are varied, including maintenance of stable extracellular ion and neurotransmitter levels, structural support, formation of extracellular matrix (ECM), modulation of synaptic function, and formation and regulation of the blood-brain barrier (BBB) (Abbott et al. 2006; Sofroniew and Vinters 2010).

Astrocytes respond to insult in the CNS through the incompletely understood phenomenon of reactive astrogliosis, which is a hallmark of all CNS pathologies, including multiple sclerosis (MS), traumatic brain injury (TBI), and spinal cord injury (SCI) (Sofroniew 2009; Sofroniew 2015b). This process entails a spectrum of potential changes in gene expression, cell structure, and astrocyte function that varies with the nature and severity of the insult (Sofroniew 2015a). Thus, reactive astrocytes may behave in a certain manner in response to a neuroinflammatory disorder such as MS, and function in a much different capacity in the case of trauma like SCI. While the implications of astrogliosis are multifaceted, the process is not a simple all-or-nothing response, rather it is a finely gradated continuum of molecular, cellular, and functional changes that range from transient alterations in gene expression and cellular hypertrophy to robust cell proliferation with compact scar formation and irreversible tissue rearrangement (**Fig. 1.1**). Different signaling mechanisms regulate different aspects of pro- or anti-inflammatory functions of reactive astrocytes, thus astrogliosis can confer both beneficial and detrimental effects in a highly context-dependent manner (Burda and Sofroniew 2014; Sofroniew 2009; Sofroniew 2014; Sofroniew 2015b; Sofroniew and Vinters 2010). Though astrogliosis is associated with many beneficial functions, under certain circumstances severe forms of the process may lead to detrimental effects, such as compact scar formation, that can inhibit the regeneration of injured neurons (Silver and Miller 2004). The notion of astrocytopathies – dysfunctions of astrocytes and astrogliosis that can contribute to or be primary causes of CNS disorders, is an area of active investigation (Sofroniew 2015b; Verkhratsky et al. 2013b; Verkhratsky et al. 2012). Reactive astrogliosis plays a fundamental role in determining tissue repair and outcome after CNS injury or disease, thus a thorough understanding of the governing molecular mechanisms is indispensable for development of therapeutic targets.

1.2   NEUROINFLAMMATION

Inflammation is a pathological hallmark of many neurodegenerative,
traumatic, and autoimmune CNS disorders. In neurodegenerative and traumatic
disorders, inflammation is locally restricted in the CNS and tends to resolve over
time, whereas in autoimmune disorders, CNS inflammation is widespread and
can be continuous or recurring (McFarland and Martin 2007). Understanding the
specific cellular mechanisms which regulate the infiltration of inflammatory cells
into the CNS during autoimmune disease is crucial to the development of
treatment strategies aiming to block continuous inflammation and improve
functional outcomes in neuroinflammatory diseases.

Astrocytes play a central role in the regulation of autoimmune CNS
inflammation, as they are intimately associated with and signal to blood vessels
(Iadecola and Nedergaard 2007) and regulate leukocyte trafficking and
inflammation in the CNS (Brosnan and Raine 2013; Rothhammer and Quintana
2015). Astrogliosis in response to inflammation is a multifaceted and context-
dependent process. Astrocytes produce many pro-inflammatory chemokines and
cytokines, as well as reactive oxygen species (ROS) *in vitro*, consistent with a
pro-inflammatory role, but also release anti-inflammatory cytokines and ROS
scavengers, thereby suggesting a role in attenuating inflammation (Dong and
Benveniste 2001; Nair et al. 2008). *In vivo*, astrocytes trigger innate pro-
inflammatory responses after CNS trauma and stroke (Farina et al. 2007; Kim et
al. 2014), while, conversely, it has been shown in numerous studies that scar-
forming reactive astrocytes form barriers essential in restricting leukocyte

migration from areas of damaged tissue into neighboring healthy tissue (Bush et

al. 1999; Faulkner et al. 2004; Herrmann et al. 2008; Li et al. 2008; Myer et al.

2006; Okada et al. 2006). Thus, astrocytes are thought to play complex roles in

regulating CNS inflammation.

1.2.1 Multiple sclerosis

Multiple sclerosis (MS) is a multifocal demyelinating neuroinflammatory

disease with progressive neurodegeneration caused by an immune response to

self-antigens in a genetically susceptible individual (Nylander and Hafler 2012).

Clinical symptoms usually begin to occur in young adults and vary based on

lesion site, often correlating with infiltration of inflammatory cells across the

blood-brain barrier (BBB), resulting in edema and demyelination (Hafler 2004).

Nearly 80% of patients present initially with a clinically isolated syndrome,

followed by a series of subacute clinical events that spontaneously abate,

referred to as relapsing remitting MS (RR-MS). While patients generally return to

near normal neurologic function at the cessation of each episode, over a variable

period of time there can be a chronic progression of clinical disability, termed

secondary progressive MS (SP-MS), which can be delayed by early therapeutic

intervention (Gunnarsson et al. 2011; Nylander and Hafler 2012). Around 15% of

patients exhibit disease progression from the start, without preceding relapses

and remissions, termed primary progressive MS (PP-MS) (Compston and Coles

2002; Miller and Leary 2007). Myelin is thought to be the primary target of

infiltrating immune cells, thus lesions consisting of areas of inflammation and

demyelination are classically located in white matter (Lassmann et al. 2007).
Axonal transection and axonal loss can occur in lesioned areas, which may
contribute to permanent disability.

MS is classically viewed as a CD4+ T cell-mediated immune disease,
whereby activated T cells recognize CNS white matter as non-self and target it
for destruction. However, a host of other peripheral immune cells and activated
CNS-resident cell populations are also involved in the course of the disease
including macrophages, microglia, oligodendrocytes, and astrocytes (McFarland
and Martin 2007; Sospedra and Martin 2005).

1.2.2 Experimental autoimmune encephalomyelitis

Experimental autoimmune encephalomyelitis (EAE) is the most widely
employed mouse model of MS and has been the major preclinical model used to
derive many current MS treatments (Croxford et al. 2011; Gold et al. 2006; Mix et
al. 2010; Ransohoff 2012; Slavin et al. 2010). Like MS, EAE is a T cell-mediated
autoimmune disease in which perivascular T cells, followed by macrophages,
enter the CNS, leading to lesioned areas of demyelination and axonal loss, which
correlates with motor deficits in standard EAE clinical scores (Herz et al. 2010;
Wujek et al. 2002). The pathology of perivascular demyelinating lesions show
similarities with human MS lesions, although the spinal cord is the primary target
in EAE whereas in MS, the brain, particularly white matter, is more often targeted
(Croxford et al. 2011; Croxford and Miyake 2016). EAE has been noted to have
strain-specific effects. For example, in SJL and Biozzi strains of mice, EAE-

induced deficits are chronic-relapsing, similar to that of RR-MS, while in C57BL/6

strain background, EAE follows a more progressive course, resembling PP-MS

or SP-MS (Croxford et al. 2011; Croxford and Miyake 2016). The basic concept

in EAE is to induce an immune response to a myelin antigen. In active EAE, an

animal is immunized with a myelin antigen along with nonspecific immune

stimulators complete Freund's adjuvant (CFA), tuberculosis bacterium (TB), and

Pertussis toxin (PTx). The simultaneous presence of a myelin antigen with

nonspecific immune stimulation leads to the identification of myelin as a non-self-

peptide and subsequent specific immune response, mimicking an autoimmune

disease like MS. The T-cells generated through this immunization regimen cross

the BBB and propagate an influx of monocytes into the CNS, with subsequent

activation of resident microglia and astrocytes, leading to demyelination of axons

and axonal transection both within and beyond these areas of immune cell

infiltration (Croxford et al. 2011; Croxford and Miyake 2016).

1.2.3 Estrogens and neuroprotection

There are significant gender differences in the prevalence of human

autoimmune diseases, including systemic lupus erythematosus (SLE),

rheumatoid arthritis (RA), Graves disease, and MS, all of which are more

prevalent in females (Spence and Voskuhl 2012). Epidemiological studies have

established that the female to male ratio for MS incidence currently ranges from

2:1 to 3:1, varying by region, and seems to have increased over the past 60

years (Voskuhl and Gold 2012). During the third trimester of pregnancy, circulating levels of estrogens are at their peak, and this correlates with a reduction in relapse rates among women with MS. Post-partum, levels of estrogens drop markedly and correlate with a significant increase in relapse rates during the 3-6 months after delivery (Confavreux et al. 1998). In addition, some studies demonstrate that pregnancy may offer long term protection to women with MS via regulation of the immune response (Runmarker and Andersen 1995; Verdru et al. 1994). This phenomenon suggests that sex hormones are important in MS disease pathogenesis and activity. In addition, while women exhibit a higher incidence of MS and a more robust immune response, male patients tend to demonstrate a more progressive disease course and higher morbidity (Dunn et al. 2015). These sex differences are also found in EAE animal models, depending on strain (Papenfuss et al. 2004).

Consistent with the clinical observations described above, it is established that estrogens are neuroprotective in numerous animal disease models of the CNS, as well as in MS. EAE in rodents improves during pregnancy and estrogen treatment exerts well-documented neuroprotective effects in EAE in both sexes of mice and multiple strains via numerous anti-inflammatory effects in the peripheral immune system (Laffont et al. 2015; Voskuhl and Gold 2012). Since estrogens are lipophilic and thus able to cross the BBB, CNS cell populations are potential estrogen targets (Wise et al. 2001). Two nuclear estrogen receptor (ER) subtypes – ERα and ERβ – are known to exist (Arevalo et al. 2015). Astrocytes express ERs (Garcia-Ovejero et al. 2002) and removal of reactive astrocytes has been reported to worsen EAE (Voskuhl et al. 2009). Interestingly, it has recently been shown that astrocytes are central players in modulating the neuroprotective effects of estrogen ligand treatment in EAE through ERα signaling and subsequent modulation of the immune response (Giraud et al. 2010; Spence et al. 2011; Spence et al. 2013), specifically through effects on CNS infiltration of T cells and phagocytic monocytes. Thus, ERα expression on astrocytes is indispensable in providing estrogen ligand-mediated neuroprotection in EAE.

1.3   VOLTAGE-GATED SODIUM CHANNELS

Voltage-gated sodium channels are heteromeric transmembrane protein complexes that are a molecular hallmark of excitable cells. Membrane depolarization triggers their activation, generating transient inward sodium currents that initiate action potentials in neurons, cardiac myocytes, and skeletal muscle cells. Sodium currents were discovered by Hodgkin and Huxley using the voltage clamp technique and reported in their groundbreaking series of papers in 1952; Catterall et al. (2005) subsequently began a molecular characterization of sodium channels from excitable membranes in the 1980's. It is now known that there are nine pore-forming α-subunits of sodium channels, Nav1.1-Nav1.9, encoded by genes *SCN1A-SCN11A* (Catterall et al. 2005), which associate with one or more non-pore-forming β-subunits encoded by *SCN1B-SCN4B* (Brackenbury and Isom 2011), lending considerable pharmacological and electrophysiological diversity, and possibly explaining their unique tissue-specific expression patterns (Catterall et al. 2005). The canonical role of these channels in driving electrogenesis and conduction in neurons (Nav1.1, Nav1.2, Nav1.3, Nav1.6, Nav1.7, Nav1.8), myocytes (Nav1.4), and cardiomyocytes (Nav1.5) has been extensively studied and is well-characterized (Catterall 2012; Waxman 2000), with a great deal of effort being put forth investigating the pathological consequences of sodium channel dysfunction in neurological disorders including neuropathic pain (Dib-Hajj et al. 2007; Dib-Hajj et al. 2013; Wood 2007), peripheral neuropathy (Faber et al. 2012a; Faber et al. 2012b; Hoeijmakers et al. 2015), epilepsy (Helbig et al. 2008; Oliva et al. 2012), multiple sclerosis

(Waxman 2006; Waxman 2008), cardiac arrhythmias such as Brugada syndrome and long QT syndrome (Liu et al. 2014; Remme 2013), and muscular disorders (Cannon 2010).

1.3.1 Noncanonical expression and role

In addition to being expressed in cells capable of generating action potentials, sodium channels have also been identified in cells that have not traditionally been considered to be electrically excitable ("nonexcitable cells"), leading to speculation as to their functional role (for review, Black and Waxman, 2013). Voltage-gated sodium channels have been documented in immune cells such as macrophages (Black et al. 2013; Carrithers et al. 2011; Carrithers et al. 2009; Carrithers et al. 2007; Schmidtmayer et al. 1994), lymphocytes (DeCoursey et al. 1985; Decoursey et al. 1987; Fraser et al. 2008; Lai et al. 2000; Lo et al. 2012), and dendritic cells (Kis-Toth et al. 2011; Zsiros et al. 2009), in addition to fibroblasts (Chatelier et al. 2012; Estacion 1991; Li et al. 2009; Munson et al. 1979), osteoblasts (Black et al. 1995b), keratinocytes (Zhao et al. 2008), epithelial cells (Wu et al. 2006; Wu et al. 2008), and others. Sodium channels contribute to multiple, varied cellular functions in these cells including phagocytosis (Carrithers et al. 2007), migration (Fraser et al. 2008; Kis-Toth et al. 2011; Wu et al. 2008), and proliferation (Wu et al. 2006). Furthermore, it is becoming increasingly recognized that the expression of sodium channels correlates with invasiveness and metastatic potential in some types of cancer cells (Patel and Brackenbury 2015; Roger et al. 2015) including prostate

(Brackenbury and Djamgoz 2006; Diss et al. 2005; Fraser et al. 2003), breast (Brackenbury et al. 2007; Driffort et al. 2014; Gillet et al. 2009; Nelson et al. 2015; Yang et al. 2012), ovarian (Gao et al. 2010), melanoma (Carrithers et al. 2009) and colon (House et al. 2010; House et al. 2015).

1.3.2. Glial expression of sodium channels

Though glia, too, are have traditionally been considered nonexcitable, multiple studies have demonstrated that these cells, including oligodendrocyte precursor (NG2[+]) cells, Schwann cells, Müller glia, microglia, and astrocytes also express voltage-gated sodium channels (**Table 1.1**). There is growing evidence that these channels regulate or participate in effector functions of glia through signaling mechanisms that are just beginning to be understood. The regulation of glial function by sodium channels has implications for the response of reactive glia to central nervous system (CNS) disease and insult.

The earliest indication of voltage-gated sodium channels in glia originated from patch-clamp studies on cultured astrocytes (Bevan et al. 1985) and Schwann cells (Chiu et al. 1984), which showed fast-activating, fast-inactivating currents that were blocked with the sodium channel-specific antagonists saxitoxin (STX) and tetrodotoxin (TTX). Patch-clamp recordings have since confirmed the expression of functional sodium channels in oligodendrocyte precursor cells (Chen et al. 2008; Karadottir et al. 2008; Kettenmann et al. 1991; Kressin et al. 1995; Linnertz et al. 2011; Sontheimer et al. 1989), Schwann cells (Howe and Ritchie 1990), microglia (Korotzer and Cotman 1992; Nicholson and Randall

2009; Persson et al. 2014), and astrocytes (Barres et al. 1988; Barres et al. 1989; Sontheimer et al. 1992; Sontheimer and Waxman 1992). Importantly, voltage-dependent sodium currents have been detected in astrocytes *in situ* within spinal cord (Chvatal et al. 1995) and hippocampal (Sontheimer and Waxman 1993) slices and in "tissue print" preparations (Barres et al. 1990). Patch clamp recordings lend the ability to distinguish between the expression of sodium channels that are sensitive to nanomolar levels of TTX (TTX-S; Nav1.1, Nav1.2, Nav1.3, Nav1.4, Nav1.5, Nav1.7) and those that require micromolar concentrations of TTX for blockade (TTX-R; Nav1.5, Nav1.8, Nav1.9), thus different VGSC alpha isoforms can be experimentally targeted via varying levels of TTX.

Microglia express a variety of voltage-gated ion channels, including sodium channels (Kettenmann et al. 2011), the predominant isoform being TTX-S Nav1.6 (**Fig. 1.2A**) (Black et al. 2009; Craner et al. 2005). Using whole-cell voltage clamp on cultured rat microglia, depolarization-induced sodium currents were elicited and then completely blocked by 0.3 µM TTX, consistent with the presence of functional TTX-S sodium channels (Persson et al. 2014) (**Fig. 1.2B-D**) and microglia within normal CNS tissues exhibit low levels of Nav1.6 immunolabeling *in situ* (Black and Waxman 2012).

In contrast to the low levels of sodium channel expression exhibited by unperturbed microglia, there is a marked upregulation of Nav1.6 in microglia within the context of experimental autoimmune encephalomyelitis (EAE), an inflammatory/demyelinating model of multiple sclerosis (MS), both at the mRNA and protein levels (**Fig. 1.2E**) (Craner et al. 2005). Intriguingly, Nav1.6

expression in reactive microglia is dynamic, with upregulated expression

corresponding to increasing disease severity of the animal and coincident with a

morphological transformation into an amoeboid appearance in microglia in both

the spinal cord and optic nerve (**Fig. 1.2F**) (Craner et al. 2005). Similarly, while

microglia from human control tissue obtained at autopsy from individuals without

neurological disease show minimal levels of Nav1.6 immunolabeling, microglia

found within active MS lesions show robust Nav1.6 expression, along with a

change in morphology from ramified to amoeboid (Craner et al. 2005).

Additionally, a recent study identified the preferential accumulation of Nav1.6

within lamellipodia of ATP-activated microglia *in vitro* (**Fig. 1.2A**) (Persson et al.

2014). Collectively, these data suggest a phenomenon of upregulated sodium

channel expression in microglia that is correlated to the extent of CNS pathology,

consistent with a functional role of sodium channels in the response of reactive

microglia to inflammation/demyelination.

In astrocytes, the TTX-R (Rogart et al. 1989) cardiac isoform Nav1.5

(Black et al. 1998; Black et al. 2010) is the predominant sodium channel

characterized, though expression of Nav1.2, Nav1.3 (Black et al. 1995a), and

Nav1.6 (Reese and Caldwell 1999) have also been reported. Black et al. (1998)

demonstrated Nav1.5 mRNA and protein in rodent astrocytes *in vitro* and *in situ*.

In parallel to microglia, the expression of sodium channels in astrocytes has been

well-documented as a dynamic process. *In vitro*, the density of sodium channels

in astrocytes varies according to culture conditions and the extracellular milieu

(Thio and Sontheimer 1993; Thio et al. 1993). Astrocytic sodium channel expression is also modulated by exposure to injury or disease. In an *in vitro* model of astrogliosis, in which a confluent monolayer of astrocytes was scratched linearly, MacFarlane and Sontheimer (1998) described a shift from TTX-S sodium currents to TTX-R sodium currents with properties attributed to Nav1.5 in response to the injury, and there was a significant increase in the numbers of scarring, proliferating astrocytes along the edges of the injury displaying transient sodium currents compared to control astrocytes (MacFarlane and Sontheimer 1997). Consistent with this earlier work, markedly upregulated expression of Nav1.5 was reported in reactive astrocytes along the borders of the injury in the same *in vitro* model (Samad et al. 2012).

Notably, Black et al. (2010) observed the upregulation of Nav1.5 on rapid-autopsy tissue, which is not seen in normal control brains, in human scarring astrocytes *in situ* within acute and chronic MS lesions (**Fig. 1.3**), surrounding new and old stroke lesions, and along the borders of CNS tumors, including gliomas and a metastatic carcinoma. Consistent with these observations, Bordey and Sontheimer (1998) reported the expression of functional sodium channels in astrocytoma cells. Finally, Nav1.5 upregulation has been observed in scarring astrocytes following a contusion spinal cord injury (SCI) (unpublished observations). Together, as in microglia, these observations suggest a commonality of upregulated astrocytic sodium channels in response to CNS tissue injury and disease and thus a possible function in reactive astrogliosis.

1.3.3 Functional role of sodium channels in glia

Microglia

Despite the long-characterized expression of sodium channels in neuroglia, their functional role (**Table 1.2**) has remained elusive until recent years. Microglia are motile resident immune cells within the brain and spinal cord that normally provide surveillance to the healthy CNS and become reactive in response to tissue insult, pathogenic challenge, or signaling within the CNS. Microgliosis involves migration, phagocytosis and secretion of chemokines, cytokines, and reactive species (Colton 2009; Hanisch and Kettenmann 2007; Ransohoff and Perry 2009). To test the notion that sodium channels modulate the microglial response to inflammation/demyelination, mice were inoculated with myelin oligodendrocyte glycoprotein (MOG 35-55) to induce EAE and fed chow supplemented with phenytoin (Lo et al. 2003), a clinically-used antiepileptic drug that blocks sodium channels (Mantegazza et al. 2010). Mice receiving phenytoin chow 10 days post-EAE induction had a four-fold decrease in the number of CD45/CD11b/c-positive microglia (Sedgwick et al. 1991) within spinal cords compared to untreated mice when assessed at 18 days (**Fig. 1.4A**), which was coincident with a significant improvement in clinical status (Craner et al. 2005). Additionally, Morsali et al. (2013) demonstrated significant axonal protection with the sodium channel blocker safinamide in EAE, even with administration delayed until the onset of clinical symptoms. Rats treated with high dose safinamide for 2 weeks showed greater numbers of surviving and functional axons than did controls treated with saline and 10% of safinamide-treated rats exhibited bilateral hindlimb paralysis at the end of the trial compared with 65% of controls, outcomes the authors partially attributed to reduced microglial/macrophage activation, and thus less production of neurotoxic reactive oxygen species (ROS) (Morsali et al. 2013).

Further investigation into the mechanisms of the beneficial effect of sodium channel blockade in EAE has demonstrated the functional role of sodium channels, particularly Nav1.6, in multiple aspects of microglial response to CNS insult including phagocytosis (Black et al. 2009; Craner et al. 2005), chemokine/cytokine release (Black et al. 2009; Morsali et al. 2013), and migration (Black et al. 2009; Persson et al. 2014). Craner et al. (2005) demonstrated that sodium channel blockade with TTX and phenytoin attenuates phagocytosis by 40% in cultured lipopolysaccharide (LPS)-stimulated microglia and demonstrated a reduction of 65% in the phagocytic ability of microglia derived from *med* mice, in which functional Nav1.6 channels are lacking (Kohrman et al. 1996), compared to microglia from wild-type mice. Black et al. (2009) additionally showed a 50-60% reduction in microglial phagocytic activity with TTX and phenytoin (**Fig. 1.4B**). Furthermore, TTX and phenytoin attenuated the release of multiple inflammatory cytokines and chemokines including interleukin 1-α (IL-1α), IL-1β and tumor necrosis factor α (TNF-α) from reactive microglia with minimal effects on IL-2, IL-4, IL-6, IL-10, monocyte chemotactic protein 1 (MCP-1; also known as CCL2), and transforming growth factor α (TGF-α), and safinamide administration reduced superoxide production and enhanced synthesis of the anti-oxidant glutathione in cultured microglia activated by phorbol-12-myristate-13-acetate (PMA) or LPS (Morsali et al. 2013). Thus, it is

plausible that sodium channel blockers have the potential to exert clinically

relevant effects in diseases such as MS through a decrease in the pro-

inflammatory microglial response.

A crucial and early functional response of reactive microglia is directed

migration to focal sites of injury or infection within the CNS, which is a complex

and highly coordinated process involving multiple cellular pathways, including

transduction of external migratory signals, membrane adhesion and retraction,

microglial polarization, and rearrangement of cytoskeletal proteins (Kettenmann

et al. 2011). Microglial chemotaxis is also associated with pathological conditions

occurring outside the CNS such as neuropathic pain (Beggs et al. 2012; Tsuda et

al. 2013; Watkins et al. 2001); thus a detailed molecular mechanisms underlying

this phenomenon may inform development of potential common therapeutic

targets for both CNS and peripheral neurological diseases. One of the initial

structural events required for migration is the formation of lamellipodia (Bisi et al.

2013), membrane protrusions containing polymerized actin (F-actin), actin-

binding proteins, Ca^{2+}-binding molecules, and the GTP-binding signaling protein

Rac (Honda et al. 2001; Ridley 1994; Ridley et al. 1992; Siddiqui et al. 2012).

Rac signaling has been identified as a crucial component in the formation of

lamellipodia (Hall 1998) and MAP kinases have been linked to reorganization of

actin filaments and cellular motility (Huang et al. 2004). Ca^{2+} signaling also plays

a critical role in lamellipodia protrusion and motility, as cell migration is Ca^{2+}-

dependent (Schwab et al. 2012; Wei et al. 2012). It is interesting to note that both

Rac1 and MAP kinase activity are modulated by levels of intracellular Ca^{2+} (Aspenstrom 2004; Chuderland et al. 2008; Price et al. 2003; Wiegert and Bading 2011).

To assess the role of sodium channel activity in the pathways leading to migration, microglia were allowed to travel toward a chemoattractant in a trans-well plate in the presence or absence of sodium channel blockers (Black et al. 2009). As seen in **Fig. 1.4C**, ATP produced an almost four-fold increase in the mean number of microglia migrating through the pores of the trans-well membrane. This cell migration was significantly reduced (~50%) in the presence of phenytoin or 0.3 µM TTX (Black et al. 2009). Recently, Persson et al. (2014) demonstrated the robust expression and preferential distribution of Nav1.6 to lamellipodia of ATP-activated microglia (**Fig. 1.5A**); the ATP-induced formation of lamellipodia is decreased (~50%) by treatment with TTX (**Fig. 1.5B**) and in *med* mice, which lack functional Nav1.6 (Persson et al. 2014). Furthermore, sodium channel blockade with 0.3 µM TTX attenuated the ATP-induced increase in levels of active Rac1 (**Fig. 1.6A**) in addition to the ATP-induced phosphorylation of MAP kinase ERK1/2 (**Fig. 1.6B**) (Persson et al. 2014). Coincident with reduced active Rac1 and phosphorylated ERK1/2 levels, TTX additionally enhanced recovery of the Ca^{2+} transient in microglia following ATP stimulation (**Fig. 1.6C**), which may explain the effects of sodium channel blockade on decreasing active Rac1 and phosphorylated ERK1/2 levels (Persson et al. 2014). Collectively, these studies demonstrate an important functional role of sodium channels in regulating the behavior of reactive microglia.

Astrocytes

The function of sodium channels in astrocytes has been unknown to date. Astrocytes serve multiple important functions in the CNS, including metabolic support of neurons, regulation of CNS ionic homeostasis, participation in formation and maintenance of the blood-brain barrier, and orchestration of the CNS response to injury and disease through astrogliosis. A standing Na^+ influx in astrocytes is necessary for Na^+/K^+-ATPase activity and Sontheimer et al. (1994) postulated that sodium channels may provide a pathway for Na^+ to enter the cell to maintain $[Na^+]_i$ at levels necessary for Na^+/K^+-ATPase activity which, in turn, supports ionic homeostasis in the CNS, particularly regarding K^+ fluxes. Furthermore, it has been reported through ^{23}Na MRI that sodium concentrations are elevated in acute and chronic MS lesions compared to normal appearing white matter (Inglese et al. 2010), which poses a possible clinical correlate to the suggestion of Black et al. (2010) that astrocytic Nav1.5 upregulation may provide a compensatory mechanism to maintain ionic homeostasis mediated by Na^+/K^+-ATPase activity within areas of CNS insult.

Along with increasing recognition of the importance of astrocytes in CNS function, views have shifted from that of astrocytes as traditionally non-excitable cells to the recognition that astrocytes exhibit excitability by way of ion fluxes, particularly in the form of $[Ca^{2+}]_i$ oscillations. Astroglial $[Ca^{2+}]_i$ fluxes are critical for numerous homeostatic cellular functions (Parnis et al. 2013; Stanimirovic et al. 1995; Wang et al. 2010). Recent work has underscored the importance of $[Na^+]_i$ fluctuations in contributing to astroglial excitability and cellular homeostasis, with a prominent mechanism involving the linkage of transmembrane movements of Na$^+$ and Ca^{2+} (Kirischuk et al. 2012; Parpura and Verkhratsky 2012; Rose and Karus 2013; Verkhratsky et al. 2013a). The reversal potential of NCX in astrocytes is set at levels close to the resting membrane potential (Reyes et al. 2012), therefore NCX can rapidly switch into reverse mode in response to small $[Na^+]_i$ increases (Kirischuk et al. 2012; Paluzzi et al. 2007), causing an increase in $[Ca^{2+}]_i$ and downstream signaling. This recent evidence supporting reverse NCX activity as a Ca^{2+} source for astrocytes suggests a potential functional role for astrocytic sodium channels as they relate to $[Ca^{2+}]_i$ fluctuations and downstream effector functions of astrocytes in the healthy and diseased CNS (Kirischuk et al. 2012; Parpura et al. 2016; Rose and Verkhratsky 2016).

1.4   SPECIFIC AIMS

The underlying goal of this thesis work was to build upon the current understanding of the presence and function of voltage-gated sodium channels (VGSCs) in glia, with a focus on astrocytes. We sought to further characterize the expression of astroglial sodium channels in neuroinflammatory diseases by looking at two mouse models of MS – one mimicking a disease like secondary-progressive MS (SP-MS) and one modeling relapsing remitting MS (RR-MS). To investigate the functional role of astroglial sodium channels, we started with an *in vitro* model of astrogliosis to explore the contribution of sodium channels to the normal functioning of astrocytes in response to injury and further investigated the underlying molecular mechanisms. Finally, we created a mouse line with a conditional astrocyte sodium channel knockout to examine the contribution of Nav1.5 in astrocytes to the course of neuroinflammatory disease *in vivo*.

Table 1.1 Voltage-gated sodium channels in glia		
Cell type	**Sodium Currents / Channels**	**References**
Astrocytes	TTX-S, TTX-R / Nav1.2, Nav1.3, Nav1.5, Nav1.6	(Barres et al. 1988; Barres et al. 1989; Bevan et al. 1985; Bevan et al. 1987; Black et al. 1998; Black et al. 2010; Black et al. 1995a; Bordey and Sontheimer 1998; Kressin et al. 1995; MacFarlane and Sontheimer 1998; Nowak et al. 1987; Reese and Caldwell 1999; Schaller et al. 1995; Sontheimer et al. 1992; Sontheimer et al. 1994; Sontheimer et al. 1991; Sontheimer and Waxman 1992; Thio and Sontheimer 1993)
Microglia	TTX-S / Nav1.1, Nav1.5, Nav1.6	(Black et al. 2009; Craner et al. 2005; Korotzer and Cotman 1992; Nicholson and Randall 2009; Norenberg et al. 1994; Persson et al. 2014; Schmidtmayer et al. 1994)
Müller glia	TTX-S, TTX-R / Nav1.6, Nav1.9	(Chao et al. 1994; Francke et al. 1996; Linnertz et al. 2011; O'Brien et al. 2008)
Oligodendrocyte precursor (NG2⁺) cells	TTX-S	(Bevan et al. 1987; Chen et al. 2008; Karadottir et al. 2008; Kettenmann et al. 1991; Kressin et al. 1995; Linnertz et al. 2011; Sontheimer et al. 1989; Tong et al. 2009; Williamson et al. 1997)
Schwann cells	TTX-S / Nav1.2, Nav1.3	(Chiu et al. 1984; Howe and Ritchie 1990; Oh et al. 1994; Schaller et al. 1995)

Table 1.2 Sodium channel functions in glia

Cell type	Effect	References
Astrocytes	TTX: attenuates Na^+/K^+-ATPase activity Veratidine: increases NOS activity	(Oka et al. 2004; Sontheimer et al. 1994)
Microglia	TTX, phenytoin: attenuate phagocytosis, migration, cytokine release TTX: attenuates lamellipodia formation, decreases active Rac-1 levels, decreases phosphorylated ERK1/2 levels, and decreases $[Ca^{2+}]_i$ response after ATP stimulation	(Black et al. 2009; Craner et al. 2005; Persson et al. 2014)
Müller glia	TTX, STX, phenytoin: inhibit ligand-induced release of glutamate	(Linnertz et al. 2011)
Oligodendrocyte precursor cells ($NG2^+$)	TTX, Nav1.x siRNA: attenuate GABA-induced migration	(Tong et al. 2009)

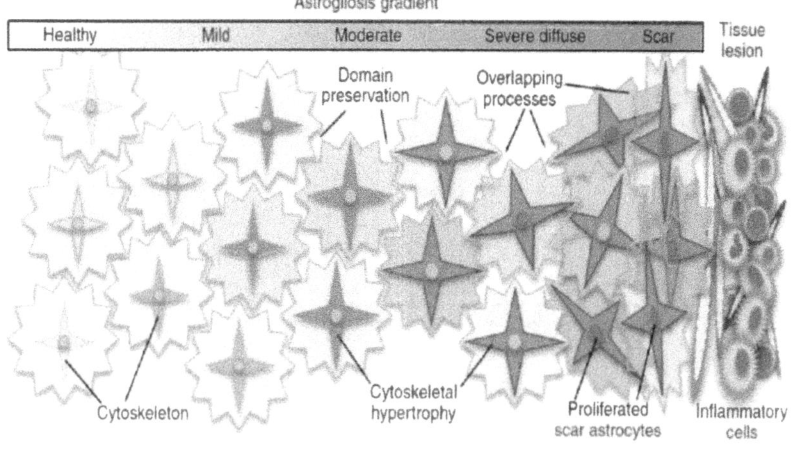

Figure 1.1 – Schema of astrogliosis from mild to moderate to scar. In healthy CNS tissue, many astrocytes do not express detectable levels of the cytoskeletal protein, GFAP. In mild to moderate astrogliosis, most astrocytes up-regulated GFAP and hypertrophy their cytoskeleton but preserve individual domains. In severe diffuse astrogliosis, this is also proliferation (depicted by red nuclei). Compact astroglial scars are comprised of newly proliferated astrocytes with densely overlapping processes that form borders to damaged tissue and inflammation. *From Sofroniew, 2015a.*

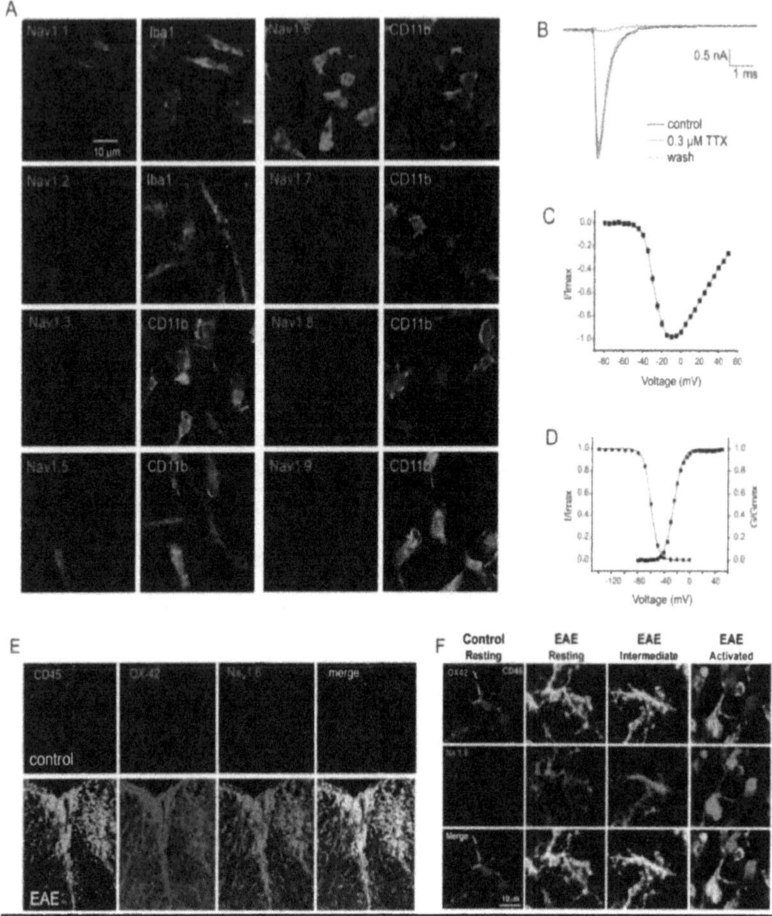

Figure 1.2 – Expression of sodium channels in microglia *in vitro* and *in vivo*. (A) Iba1+ and CD11b+ (green) microglia exhibit immunolabeling for sodium channels Nav1.1, Nav1.5, and Nav1.6 (red). Microglial exhibit background levels of Nav1.2, Nav1.3, Nav1.7, Nav1.8, and Nav1.9 immunoreactivity. [Modified from Black et al. (2009)]. **(B)** Representative sodium current traces recorded from microglial before (black) and after (red) treatment of 0.3 µM TTX. **(C)** Normalized peak current-voltage relationship. **(D)** Voltage-dependence of activation and steady-state fast-inactivation. [Modified from Persson et al. (2014)]. **E.** Images of spinal cord sections from control mice immunolabeled with CD45 (green), OX-42 (blue), and Nav1.6 (red) antibodies exhibit a lack of CD45/OX-42 immunopositive cells in control tissue (top panels). Images of spinal cord sections from EAE mice show extensive infiltration of CD45 (green) and OX-42 (blue) positive cells in EAE spinal cord, with extensive co-localization of Nav1.6 and OX-42 (yellow) and Nav1.6, OX-42, and CD45 (white) in merged image of EAE spinal cord (bottom panels). **(F)** Microglia labeled with OX-42 (blue) and CD45 (green) in control spinal cord exhibit a non-activated morphology (top row, left) and low levels of Nav1.6 immunolabeling (middle, left). In spinal cords of mice with EAE, there is a progressive transformation to an amoeboid-like appearance consistent with a phagocytic microglial phenotype (top, right) and an incremental increase in Nav1.6 immunoreactivity (middle, right). [Modified from Craner et al. (2005)]. *Data generated by JA Black, AK Persson, MJ Craner.*

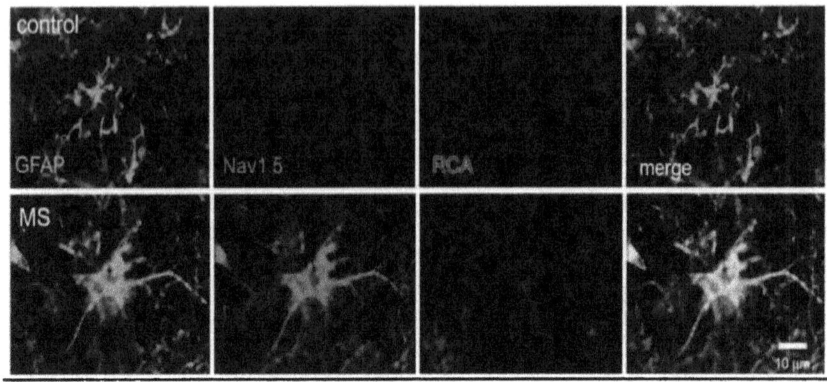

Figure 1.3 – Nav1.5 expression in astrocytes within control and multiple sclerosis lesion. GFAP-positive astrocyte (green) within control human tissue obtained at autopsy does not exhibit Nav1.5 labeling. In contrast reactive astrocyte within an active MS lesion displays robust Nav1.5 immunolabeling (red). Ricinus communis agglutinin I (RCA) positive macrophages (blue) are present adjacent to the reactive astrocyte (bottom, right). Scale bar, 10 μm. [Modified from Black et al. (2010)]. *Data generated by JA Black.*

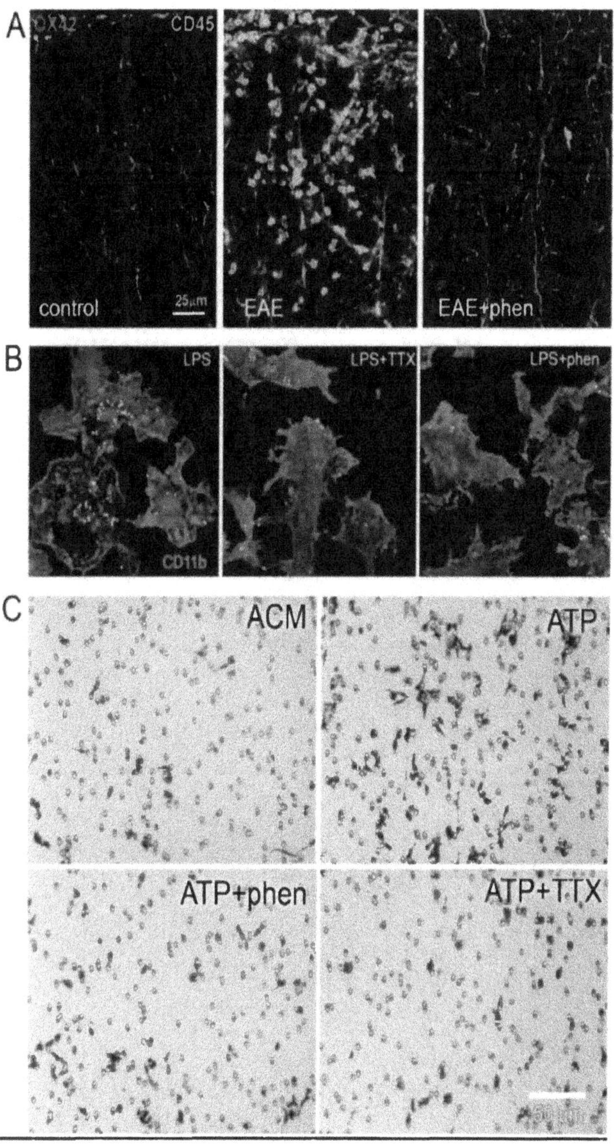
A
OX42
CD45
control
25µm
EAE
EAE+phen
B
LPS
LPS+TTX
LPS+phen
CD11b
C
ACM
ATP
ATP+phen
ATP+TTX

Figure 1.4 – Sodium channel blockade reduces effector functions of microglia. (A) Spinal cords from control, EAE, and phenytoin-treated EAE mice were immunostained with anti-CD45 (green) and anti-OX-42 (blue) antibodies. There is a notable increase in the number of immune cells within spinal cords from mice with EAE (middle) compared to control (left), and mice treated with phenytoin (right) exhibit a marked reduction of inflammatory infiltrate. [Modified from Craner et al. (2005)]. **(B)** LPS-stimulated microglia (red) exhibit marked phagocytosis of fluorescent-labeled latex beads (yellow) which is attenuated by incubation with 0.3 µm TTX and phenytoin (phen). **(C)** Microglia exhibit limited migration through the trans-well membrane in astrocyte-conditioned medium (ACM) only; in contrast, ATP stimulates many microglia to migrate which is attenuated by both phenytoin and 0.3 µM TTX. [Modified from Black et al. (2009)]. *Data generated by MJ Craner and JA Black.*

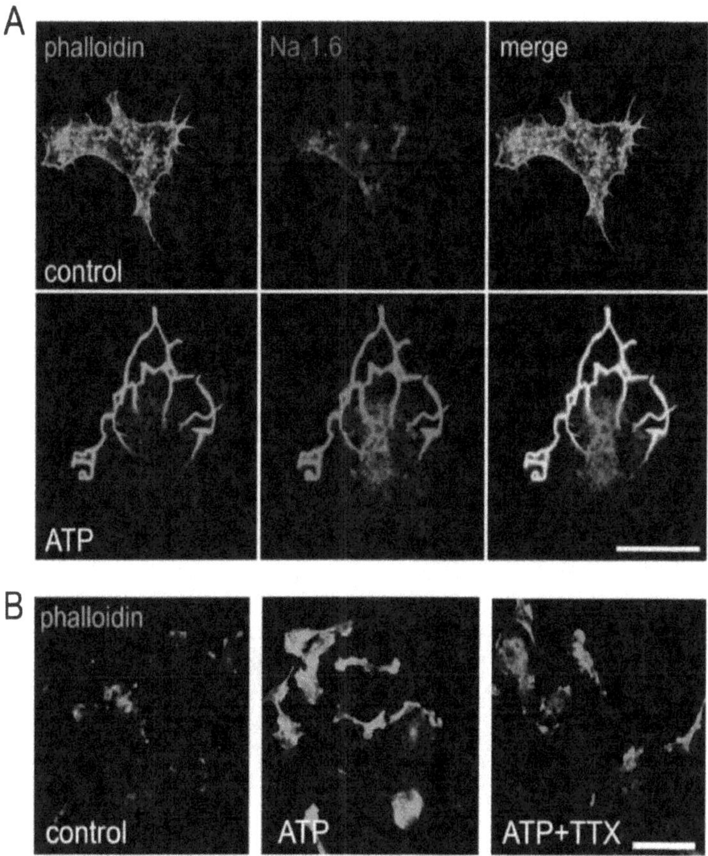

Figure 1.5 – Sodium channels contribute to lamellipodia formation in ATP-stimulated microglia. (A) Nonstimulated microglia exhibit a diffuse distribution of phalloidin (green), indicating lack of organized lamellipodia formation, and Nav1.6 (red) immunolabeling whereas ATP stimulation of microglia induces formation of lamellipodia that display robust immunolabeling for phalloidin and Nav1.6. Scale bar, 10 μm. **(B)** Nonstimulated microglia from wild-type mice display limited formation of lamellipodia (green) whereas ATP stimulation induces substantial lamellipodia formation. Treatment of ATP-stimulated microglia with 0.3 μm TTX significantly attenuates lamellipodia formation. Scale bars, 25 μm. [Modified from Persson et al. (2014)]. *Data generated by JA Black and AK Persson.*

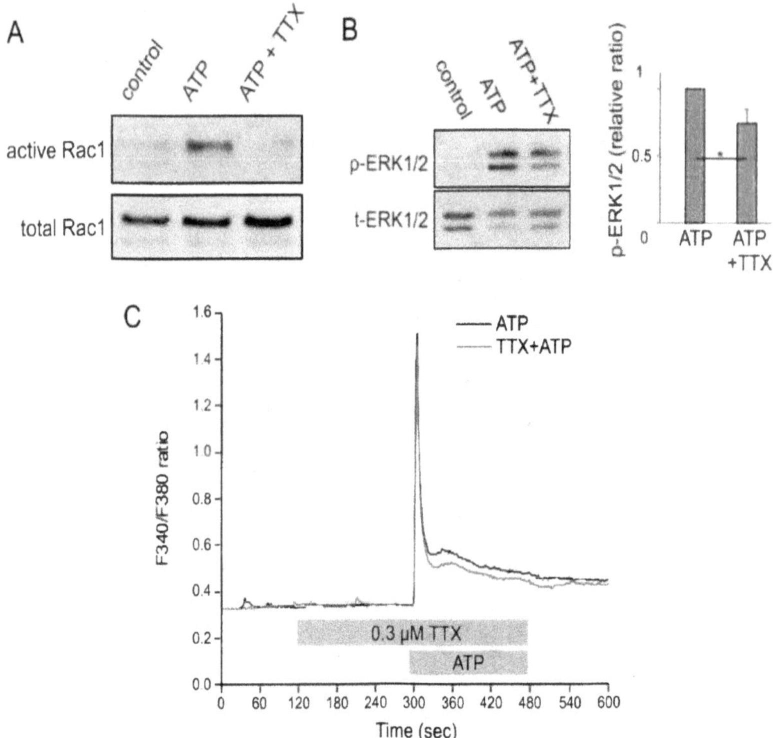

Figure 1.6 – Sodium channels contribute to Rac1 and ERK1/2 activation and [Ca^{2+}]$_i$ response in ATP-stimulated microglia. (A) A pull-down assay using the microglial cell line C8-B4 demonstrates that ATP induces elevated levels of activated Rac1 which is attenuated by 0.3 µM TTX. **(B)** Western blot analysis demonstrates that ATP stimulation of microglia increases levels of phosphorylated ERK1/2 compared to unstimulated control microglia. Treatment of ATP-activated microglia with 0.3 µM TTX significantly reduces activation of ERK1/2. **(C)** ATP stimulation induces a robust microglial [Ca^{2+}]$_i$ response (black); the recovery of the [Ca^{2+}] transient is enhanced by pretreatment with 0.3 µM TTX (red). Lines represent the ratio of fluorescent signals induced by 340 and 380 nm excitation in cells loaded with Fura-2 AM. [Modified from Persson et al. (2014)]. *Data generated by JA Black and AK Persson.*

<u>CHAPTER 2</u>: FUNCTIONAL ROLE OF NAV1.5 IN ASTROGLIOSIS IN VITRO

This chapter contains a modified version of material that appeared in the author's

publication: Pappalardo LW, Samad OA, Black JA, Waxman SG (2014). Voltage-

gated sodium channel Nav1.5 contributes to astrogliosis in an in vitro model of

glial injury via reverse Na+/Ca2+ exchange. GLIA 62:1162-1175.

2.1   INTRODUCTION

Astrocytes outnumber neurons in the brain and spinal cord and respond to

insult in the CNS through the incompletely understood process of reactive

astrogliosis, which is a hallmark of the response to injury in many CNS

pathologies. While the functional ramifications of astrogliosis are complex, recent

studies suggest that astrocytes can exert both beneficial and detrimental effects,

the outcome of which is determined by specific signaling cascades involved

(Sofroniew 2009), temporal sequence (Rolls et al. 2009), and extent and type of

injury, which determine reactive astrocyte phenotype (Zamanian et al. 2012).

Astrocytes exert many effects crucial to the healing of the CNS following injury,

as scar-forming astrocytes form barriers to protect healthy tissue from

inflammation in neighboring damaged tissue and play an important role in

reformation and maintenance of the blood-brain barrier (BBB) (Sofroniew 2015a)

However, astrocytes also exert pro-inflammatory effects through the release of

cytokines and chemokines and formation of both a physical and chemical barrier

to axon regeneration (Silver and Miller 2004; Sofroniew 2014). Thus, astrogliosis

can be regarded as a continuum; however, once the process approaches the severe end of the spectrum, the formation of a scar is long-lasting and can inhibit the regeneration of injured neurons (Sofroniew 2009; Tom et al. 2004).

Along with increasing recognition of the importance of astrocytes in CNS pathology, the past 20 years have seen a paradigm shift from the view of astrocytes as traditionally non-excitable cells to the recognition that astrocytes exhibit excitability by way of ionic fluxes, and particularly in the form of $[Ca^{2+}]_i$ oscillations. Astrocytes have a complex morphology, with a network of ultrathin and connected filaments extending to and enwrapping excitatory synapses, a structure known as the 'tripartite synapse' (Papouin et al. 2017). It has been estimated in rodents that up to 30-60% of neuronal synapses are enwrapped by astrocytes processes (Bernardinelli et al. 2014; Reichenbach et al. 2010). Astroglial $[Ca^{2+}]_i$ fluxes lead to activation of secretory machinery and exocytosis of neurotransmitters, which can modulate these neuronal synapses, a phenomenon that has been termed 'gliotransmission' (Agulhon et al. 2008). Astrocytic processes possess signaling machinery, including SNARE proteins regulating vesicular fusion and neurotransmitters such as glutamate, GABA, adenosine/ATP, and D-serine. Thus, by directly sensing neuronal activity, astrocytes participate in synaptic transmission by releasing 'gliotransmitters' that act directly on pre- or post-synaptic neuronal receptors and impact synaptic efficacy, potency, or plasticity (Papouin et al. 2017).

Aside from modulation of synaptic transmission, levels of intracellular Ca^{2+} are critical for numerous homeostatic cellular functions in astrocytes, including migration and proliferation (Parnis et al. 2013; Stanimirovic et al. 1995; Wang et al. 2010). Cytoplasmic Ca^{2+} levels in astrocytes are derived from multiple compartments, including endoplasmic reticulum (Kastritsis et al. 1992), mitochondrial sodium-calcium exchange (Parnis et al. 2013), and the extracellular space (Gao et al. 2013). One important mechanism by which $[Ca^{2+}]_i$ can be regulated in astrocytes is by reverse (Ca^{2+}-importing) activity of sodium-calcium exchangers (NCX) (Paluzzi et al. 2007; Reyes et al. 2012), the three isoforms of which are expressed in astrocytes (Minelli et al. 2007).

Recent work has also indicated the importance of $[Na^+]_i$ fluctuations in contributing to astroglial excitability and cellular homeostasis, with a prominent mechanism involving the linkage of transmembrane movements of Na^+ and Ca^{2+} (Kirischuk et al. 2012; Parpura and Verkhratsky 2012; Rose and Karus 2013). Glutamate receptors and purinoceptors, as well as voltage-gated sodium channels (VGSCs), are known to play a role in astrocytic Na^+ influx, but the molecular mechanisms controlling cytosolic Na^+ concentrations remain poorly understood (Parpura and Verkhratsky 2012). Evidence supporting reverse NCX activity as a Ca^{2+} source for astrocytes suggests a potential functional role for astrocytic sodium channels as they relate to $[Ca^{2+}]_i$ fluctuations (Kirischuk et al. 2012). Astrocytes express VGSCs (Pappalardo et al. 2016), and in particular the cardiac isotype Nav1.5 (Black et al. 1998; Black et al. 2010; MacFarlane and Sontheimer 1998). The functions of VGSCs in astrocytes, which are traditionally considered to be non-excitable, have remained elusive, although Sontheimer et al. (1994) have suggested that these channels provide a pathway for Na^+ to enter the cell to maintain $[Na^+]_i$ at levels necessary for Na^+/K^+-ATPase activity (Sontheimer 1994).

We present here, evidence supporting a contribution of sodium channel Nav1.5 to astrogliosis in an *in vitro* model of glial mechanical injury. We further implicate fluctuations in $[Ca^{2+}]_i$ due to reverse operation of NCX, triggered by VGSC activity, as the mechanism by which Nav1.5 contributes to the response of astrocytes to mechanical injury. Our results establish a link between the activity of VGSCs and astrogliosis by way of alterations in $[Ca^{2+}]_i$.

2.2   MATERIALS AND METHODS

2.2.1 Cell Culture

Cells used in all experiments were purified rat primary cortical astrocytes

from E19 Sprague-Dawley rats of mixed sexes (Invitrogen, Grand Island, NY),

which were thawed and maintained per manufacturer's recommendations. The

cells were plated on either glass coverslips in 24-well plates (Corning,

Tewksbury, MA) or 35 mm glass bottom dishes (MatTek, Ashland, MA) at a

seeding density of ~2 x 10^4 cells. Cells were grown until confluent in astrocyte

medium [Dulbecco's modified Eagle's medium +4.5 g/L D-glucose, +L-glutamine,

+110 mg/L sodium pyruvate (Invitrogen) supplemented with 15% fetal bovine

serum (Hyclone, Rockford, IL), penicillin (100 U/ml) and streptomycin (100 µg/ml)

(Invitrogen)]. Greater than 90% of cells in these cultures were GFAP-positive.

2.2.2 Immunocytochemistry

Astrocytes were fixed for 10 min in PFA solution [4% paraformaldehyde

(Sigma, St. Louis, MO) in 0.14 M Sorensen's phosphate buffer, pH 7.4], rinsed 3

times, then incubated in blocking solution [phosphate-buffered saline with 3% fish

gelatin, 0.3% Triton X-100, and 3% normal donkey serum (all from Sigma)] for 15

min at room temperature. Astrocytes were then incubated with primary antibodies

[mouse anti-glial fibrillary acidic protein (GFAP), 1:1000, Covance, Princeton, NJ;

rabbit anti-Nav1.5, 1:100, Alomone, Jerusalem, Israel] for 2-3 h at room

temperature, rinsed 3 times with phosphate-buffered saline (PBS) and incubated

with secondary antibodies [donkey anti-mouse immunoglobulin G-Alexa Fluor

488, 1:1000, Invitrogen; donkey anti-rabbit immunoglobulin G Cy3, 1:500, Jackson ImmunoResearch, West Grove, PA] for 1-2 h at room temperature. Astrocytes were rinsed with PBS and mounted with Aqua Poly mount (Polysciences, Warrington, PA). Control experiments were performed with the omission of the primary antibodies and only background labeling was observed. For Nav1.5/GFAP stained astrocytes, multiple images were acquired with a Nikon C1si confocal microscope (Nikon USA, Melville, NY) operating with frame lambda (sequential) mode and saturation indicator activated to prevent possible bleed-through between channels.

2.2.3 Scratch wound

As an *in vitro* model of the response of astrocytes to injury we used a scratch wound assay. Astrocytes were plated on glass coverslips in 24-well plastic plates. When confluent, medium was replaced with astrocyte medium (control), astrocyte medium + 10 µM TTX (Calbiochem, San Diego, CA), or astrocyte medium + 0.5 µM KB-R7943 (Calbiochem). The medium was then removed and saved while the astrocytes were mechanically scratched with a pipette tip similar to previous descriptions (Kornyei et al. 2000; MacFarlane and Sontheimer 1997; Yu et al. 1993), yielding a linear cell-free wound. Post-scrape, the cells were not washed, and saved medium was replaced in each well to continue pharmacological treatment through the duration of the assay. Cells were incubated under usual conditions for 24 h.

For experiments in which the scratched astrocytes were incubated with TTX for only the initial 15 min or 2 hour period, cells were rinsed three times with PBS after treatment with TTX for the appropriate period and incubated with astrocyte medium for the duration of the 24 h experiment.

To investigate the contribution of $[Ca^{2+}]_i$ in response to mechanical injury, the Ca^{2+} chelator Oregon-Green 488 BAPTA-AM (OGB) (Invitrogen) was employed. OGB is cleaved by cellular esterases into its active, Ca^{2+}-chelating form and the subsequent negative charge renders it trapped intracellularly. Thus, OGB chelates any intracellular $[Ca^{2+}]_i$ it encounters. Cells were incubated with 10 µM OGB with 0.125% pluronic (Invitrogen) in astrocyte medium for 1 h prior to scratch. Twenty-four hours following the mechanical injury, the cells were fixed and processed for detection of GFAP.

2.2.4 Mechanical injury quantitation

To measure the extent of wound closure in the experimental conditions, montages of the entire coverslip were obtained with a Nikon Ti-E inverted microscope (Tokyo, Japan), using a 10× objective. NIS-Elements AR software (Nikon USA, Melville, NY) was used for analysis of the average wound width (µm) of each scratched coverslip by measuring the total area of the cell-free wound and dividing by the length of the major axis. Average wound width in experimental conditions was normalized to the untreated condition for each experiment, to account for variability between cultures. For each experiment, the growth into the initial injury area at t=24 h was calculated as a percentage of the mean initial width of the wound (t=0).

To assay the consistency of the mechanical scratch, coverslips (n=31) were scratched, fixed at t=0, processed for GFAP immunocytochemistry, and imaged; the mean ± SEM initial scratch width was 414 ± 12 µm, indicating consistent initial injury.

2.2.5 Nav1.5 siRNA knockdown scratch wound

Accell siRNA molecules (pool of 4 different sequences, SMARTpool E-089491-00-0005) targeting rat Nav1.5, as well as non-targeting (NT) control Accell siRNA #1 (D- 001910-01-05) were purchased from Thermoscientific (USA) and used at a final concentration of 1 µM according to the manufacturer's protocol. Briefly, siRNA molecules were re-suspended in siRNA buffer (Thermoscientific, USA) and then added to Accell medium to a final concentration of 1 µM. Growth medium was removed from confluent astrocytes and the siRNAs or control medium (two treatment conditions: NT-siRNA in Accell medium and Nav1.5 siRNA in Accell medium) added to cells for 48 h prior to initiation of mechanical injury as described above. Standard cell lysis techniques were then used, and the RNA extracted (Samad et al. 2013). Due to variability between cultures, we normalized the results of the wound healing assay to NT siRNA, where there is minimal Nav1.5 knockdown (**Fig. 3A**).

2.2.6 Quantitative RT-PCR

Cultured rat primary cortical astrocytes were processed for RNA extraction using RNasy Microkit (Qiagen, Valencia, CA) according to the manufacturer's protocol. Three hundred ng of total RNA was used to generate 1st strand cDNA using Superscript III (Invitrogen) according to the manufacturer's protocol. Real-time Taqman PCR assays for rat: Nav1.1 (assay id: Rn00578439_m1), Nav1.2 (Rn00680558_m1), Nav1.3 (Rn01485332_m1), Nav1.4 (Rn01461132_m1), Nav1.5 (Rn00565502_m1), Nav1.6 (Rn00570506_m1), Nav1.7 (Rn00591020_m1), Nav1.8 (Rn00568393_m1), Nav1.9 (Rn00570487_m1), NCX1 (Rn00570527_m1), NCX2 (Rn00589573_m1), NCX3 (Rn01517855_m1) and rat GAPDH (Rn01775763_g1) were used with Universal Taqman PCR master mix (20×) (all from Applied Biosystems, Carlsbad, CA). One microliter of the cDNA was used as a template in 20 µl and the reaction was run in duplicates according to the manufacturer's instructions using the Eppendorf realplex (USA). Normalization and expression analysis of gene of interest mRNA were done using the 2–δCt method with GAPDH as the control.

2.2.7 Astrocyte migration assay

Astrocytes were plated in 24-well glass bottom dishes and incubated with astrocyte medium, astrocyte medium + 10 µM TTX, or astrocyte medium + 0.5 µM KB-R7943 prior to performing a scrape injury with a cell scraper. After injury, cells were transferred to an incubation chamber on a Nikon Ti-E inverted microscope (Tokyo, Japan). Phase-contrast images of the entire coverslip were obtained at multiple time points over a 24 h period, using a 10× objective. NIS-Elements AR software (Nikon USA, Melville, NY) was used for analysis of the average process extension of each coverslip (μm) by measuring process extension of individual astrocytes from original site of injury. Migration in experimental conditions was normalized to the untreated condition for each experiment, to account for variability between cultures.

2.2.8 Nav1.5 siRNA knockdown migration assay

ON-TARGET plus siRNA molecules (pool of 4 different sequences, SMARTpool L-089491-02) targeting rat Nav1.5 as well as non-targeting control #1 (D-001810-01-05) were purchased from Thermoscientific (USA) and used at a final concentration of 25 nM according to the manufacturer's protocol. Briefly, siRNA molecules were re-suspended in siRNA buffer (Thermoscientific, USA) and then added to Opti-MEM I Reduced Serum Medium (Invitrogen). Separately, Lipofectamine 2000 (Invitrogen) was added to Opti-MEM I Reduced Serum Medium and allowed to incubate for 5 min at RT. The siRNA mixture was then added to the Lipofectamine 2000 mixture and incubated for 20 min at RT. Astrocyte media was removed and delivery media (NT-siRNA/Lipofectamine 2000/Opti-MEM I medium or Nav1.5 siRNA/Lipofectamine 2000/Opti-MEM I medium) was added to the cells overnight. The cells were washed, and the delivery media was replaced with astrocyte media and cells incubated for an additional 24 h prior to initiation of the scrape injury.

2.2.9 Astrocyte proliferation assay

BrdU assays were performed to assess cell proliferation per manufacturer's instructions (Sigma). Briefly, control (no mechanical injury) and mechanically scratched astrocytes were incubated with 10 µM BrdU in astrocyte medium. After 24 h, astrocytes were fixed with PFA solution for 15 min, washed three times with PBS, permeabilized with 0.3% Triton X-100 at RT for 15 min, incubated with 2 M HCL at 37° C for 30 min, neutralized with 0.1 M borate buffer (pH=8.5) three times, and washed three times with PBS. The cells were then incubated in 500 µl PBS/3% normal donkey serum/2% fish gelatin/0.1% Triton X-100 at 37° C for 30 min, incubated with mouse anti-BrdU (1:200, Serotec) and rabbit anti-GFAP (1:1000, Chemicon, Billerica, MA) at 37° C for 30 min, washed three times with PBS, and incubated with donkey anti-mouse immunoglobulin G Cy3 (1:500, Jackson) and donkey anti-rabbit immunoglobulin G Alexa Fluor 488 (Invitrogen) at 37° C for 30 min. The cells were washed five times with PBS and mounted on slides with Aqua Poly mount.

To test the effect of TTX and KB-R7943 on proliferation, the entire procedure was repeated in the presence of these reagents for 24 h. We attempted to assess proliferation following knockdown of Nav1.5 with siRNA, but the astrocytes were not viable following transfection with siRNA plus exposure to BrdU (24 h), and thus proliferation could not be assessed.

To count BrdU-positive cells, NIS-Elements AR software was employed. A 3-5 mm^2 area was assayed for each coverslip, with the analyzed area for scratched coverslips <500 µm from the edge of the wound. The cell-free wound area was subtracted from the total area assayed and data converted to BrdU-positive cells per mm^2, both along the margin of the wound and in unscratched conditions. Each experimental condition was expressed as % proliferation compared to the value for a paired control (unscratched) at 24 h for each experiment to account for variability between cultures.

2.2.10 Measurement of $[Ca^{2+}]_i$ after injury

Astrocytes were maintained in 35 mm glass bottom dishes. Once confluent, cells were loaded with 5 µM Fura-2 AM (Invitrogen) in standard bath solution (SBS; 140 mM NaCl, 3 mM KCl, 1 mM $MgCl_2$, 1 mM $CaCl_2$, 10 mM HEPES, pH 7.3, 320 mOsm) with 0.05% pluronic (Invitrogen) at room temperature for 90 min. For cells in TTX or KB-R7943 treatment conditions, the pharmacologic agents were included in the Fura-2 AM SBS solution. After incubation, cells were rinsed twice with SBS and 2 ml SBS was placed in the dish for the remainder of the experiment. For cells in TTX or KB-R7943 treatment conditions, the pharmacologic agents were included in the 2 ml SBS placed for the duration of the experiment. Cells from a single field per dish were initially imaged with bright-field optics with a Nikon Ti-E inverted microscope. Subsequently, using a NIKON UV-2E/C filter cube with the excitation filter removed, cells were illuminated at 340 and 380 nm using filters installed in a fast wavelength switching light source (Lambda DG-4, Sutter Instruments, Novato, CA). The dichroic mirror used was 400 nm LP with a 460/50 bandpass emission filter. Images were captured with a QuantEM CCD camera (Princeton

Instruments, Trenton, NJ), and digitized with NIS- Elements AR software (Nikon). 340/380 ratio images were collected every 2 s during the experiments.

To induce mechanical injury in the cultures, cells were scratched in place with a custom quartz injury device. Astrocytes within 50 µm of the scratch edge (~3-4 cells deep) were analyzed using NIS-Elements AR software. Cells were grouped in 50 µm wide laminae due to the synchronous nature of the $[Ca^{2+}]_i$ wave traveling through the syncytium. For each experiment, 10 cells were randomly picked in each lamina utilizing bright-field optics and data for emission following 340 nm and 380 nm excitation were extracted for each region of interest (ROI). Data were background corrected based on levels in the cell-free area at the end of each experiment, after the wound had been initiated. A 340/380 ratio was manually computed for each cell along every time point during the experiment. To normalize all experiments performed on different days, the control basal level for each set of experiments was adjusted to a ratio of 0 and the treated conditions were adjusted by the same value.

2.2.11 Nav1.5 siRNA knockdown $[Ca^{2+}]_i$ measurement after injury

ON-TARGET plus siRNA molecules (pool of 4 different sequences, SMARTpool L-089491-02) targeting rat Nav1.5 mRNA as well as non-targeting control #1 (D-001810-01-05) were purchased from Thermoscientific (USA) and used at a final concentration of 25 nM according to the manufacturer's protocol and as described earlier. Delivery media (NT-siRNA/Lipofectamine 2000/Opti-MEM I medium or Nav1.5 siRNA/Lipofectamine 2000/Opti-MEM I medium) was added to the cells overnight. The cells were washed, and the delivery medium was replaced with astrocyte media and cells incubated for an additional 24 h prior to initiation of Fura-2 AM measurements as described above. After completion of the $[Ca^{2+}]_i$ measurements, standard cell lysis techniques were then used, and the RNA extracted (Samad et al. 2013).

2.2.12 Statistics

Data are presented as mean ± SEM from n determinations as indicated. Data were analyzed with an unpaired Student t-test or a one-way ANOVA (for >2 groups) followed by Tukey's honest significance test. $p < 0.05$ was considered to be a significant difference. All statistics were performed with Origin 9.0 (Origin Lab Corporation, Northampton, MA), with the exception of AUC data for $[Ca^{2+}]_i$ experiments, which was analyzed with GraphPad Prism (La Jolla, CA).

2.3   RESULTS

2.3.1 Astrocytes express Nav1.5 and NCX1

Previous studies have reported the expression of Nav1.1, Nav1.2, Nav1.3
(Black et al. 1994), Nav1.6 (Reese and Caldwell 1999), and notably Nav1.5
sodium channels (Black et al. 1998) in rodent astrocytes. Consistent with these
previous studies, we found that rat primary cortical astrocytes *in vitro* express
sodium channel Nav1.5 as evidenced by both immunocytochemical (**Fig. 2.1A**)
and RT-PCR (**Fig. 2.1B**) assays. Nav1.5 mRNA expression in astrocytes was
robust and significantly greater than that of other VGSC subtypes. Additionally,
since it is known that sodium channel activity can drive reverse Na^+/Ca^{2+}
exchange in astrocytes (Kirischuk et al. 2012; Paluzzi et al. 2007), we assessed
the expression of NCX1, NCX2, and NCX3 in the cultured cortical astrocytes by
RT-PCR and observed strong expression of NCX1 mRNA (**Fig. 2.1B**).

2.3.2 TTX and KB-R7943 inhibit astroglial response to injury

To evaluate the contribution of Nav1.5 and NCX1 in the response of
astrocytes following a scratch injury, we first took a pharmacological approach
and studied the effect of VGSC blocker (TTX) and NCX inhibitor 2-[2-[4-(4-
Nitrobenzyloxy)phenyl]ethyl]isothiourea mesylate (KB- R7943) on the response
of astrocytes to physical injury (**Fig. 2.2A**). Since Nav1.5 is resistant to block by
nanomolar levels of TTX (Rogart et al. 1989), we used a TTX concentration of 10
µM, which is known to block Nav1.5 (Catterall et al. 2005; Gu et al. 1997). A KB-
R7943 concentration of 0.5 µM was used, as the reverse mode of NCX is
selectively affected at this low dose [IC_{50} = 1.1- 3.4 µmol/L for reverse mode and

$IC_{50} > 30$ µmol/L for forward mode (Iwamoto et al. 1996; Persson et al. 2013a; Persson et al. 2013b)]. Twenty-four hours following mechanical injury by sterile pipette tip (scratch), astrocytes extended into the injury gap, resulting in 54 ± 3% (n=29) closure of the gap compared to the original wound size (t=0) (**Fig. 2.2B, C**). Upon addition of TTX, the degree of closure of the gap was attenuated, with blockade of sodium channels resulting in significantly decreased closure of 28 ± 5% of the initial gap area at t=0 (n=15, p=0.00002). Similarly, addition of KB-R7943 inhibited closure of the wound area; regrowth after 24 h was 36 ± 6% of the original wound area (n=6, p=0.03698) (**Fig. 2.2B, C**).

To determine whether the inhibitory action of TTX and KB-R7943 was additive, the effect of combined exposure to TTX + KB-R7943 compared to TTX alone was tested in separate experiments. A significant difference between TTX + KB-R7943 and TTX treatments with respect to wound closure was not detected after 24 h (data not shown), consistent with a common pathway for the effects of TTX and KB-R7943 on the response of astrocytes to mechanical injury.

We next determined whether there was a crucial time-frame for the treatment with TTX to inhibit wound closure. In separate experiments, TTX was applied for 15 min (n=5) or 2 h (n=6) after scratch and compared to TTX applied for the full 24 h period (n=5). After 24 h, there were significant differences between the degree of wound closure for control (54 ± 5%, n=7) and TTX treatment for 15 min (31 ± 5%, n=5), 2 h (31 ± 5%, n=6), and 24 h (30 ± 7%, n=5) (p=0.03740, p=0.02691, and p=0.02668, respectively), compared to original wound size at t=0, but not among the three TTX treatment groups (**Fig. 2.2D**).

These findings are consistent with an early role of VGSCs in the response of astroglia in wound closure after injury.

2.3.3 Nav1.5 knockdown inhibits astrocyte response to injury

The marked inhibition by 10 µM TTX of the glial response to mechanical injury and our finding that Nav1.5 is the predominant VGSG expressed in cultured rat cortical astrocytes obtained at E19, strongly suggest that the Nav1.5 isotype contributes to the glial response to injury *in vitro*. To demonstrate the involvement of Nav1.5, we took a loss-of- function knockdown approach using a pool of 4 specific siRNA sequences targeting the Nav1.5 mRNA. Nav1.5 knockdown after siRNA treatment was confirmed by quantitative real-time PCR, which showed that Nav1.5 mRNA expression of cells treated with Nav1.5 siRNA was significantly decreased by 70 ± 11% compared to non-targeting (NT) siRNA (p=0.01252), indicating successful knockdown of Nav1.5 (**Fig. 2.3A**). To confirm the specificity of the Nav1.5 siRNA cocktail on Nav1.5 mRNA expression, we performed real-time PCR. Minimal effects of NT siRNA or Nav1.5 siRNA treatment on the expression of Nav1.2, Nav1.6 and Nav1.7 mRNA were observed (**Fig. 2.3B**).

Due to variability between cultures, we normalized the results of the wound healing assay to NT siRNA, where there is minimal Nav1.5 knockdown (**Fig. 2.3A**). Twenty-four hours after the scratch injury, we found that exposure to Nav1.5 siRNA (n=6) reduced the amount of wound closure to 45 ± 15% compared to NT siRNA (n=6, p=0.01346) (**Fig. 2.3C, D**).

2.3.4 Astrocyte response to injury is due to migration and proliferation and both processes are attenuated by TTX and KB-R7943

Previous studies have shown that astrogliosis *in vivo* involves cell proliferation and elongation of cell processes (Faulkner et al. 2004; Wanner et al. 2013). To determine the cellular processes contributing to scratch wound closure in our experiments, we first assessed the presence of migrating cells after injury using live imaging microscopy. After a scrape-induced injury (**Fig. 2.4A**, boundary of initial injury indicated by red line), cell process extension was observed throughout the 24 h period. After 24 h, cell processes had migrated 136 ± 20 µm from the site of injury in control conditions. Compared to controls (n=9), treatment with TTX decreased this migration by 21 ± 3% (n=3, p=0.04708) and treatment with KB- R7943 decreased migration by 30 ± 6% (n=5, p=0.00256) (**Fig. 2.4B**). Similarly, astrocytes treated with NT siRNA (n=4) migrated 143 ± 6 µm from the site of injury. Treatment with Nav1.5 siRNA decreased this 24 h migration by 20 ± 7% (n=3, p= 0.04534) (**Fig. 2.4C**)

To determine whether cell proliferation contributed to wound closure, we used a BrdU assay. After 24 h, there was a significant 77 ± 9% increase in proliferation amongst cells along the edge of a scratch (n=7) compared to cells in unscratched cultures (n=8, p=0.000006) (**Fig. 2.5A, B**). Additionally, while neither TTX nor KB-R7943 affected rates of cell proliferation in cultures without a scratch compared to untreated cultures (data not shown), both agents significantly decreased proliferation of cells along the edges of a wound. Compared to untreated scratched cultures, TTX decreased proliferation by 54 ± 4%

(p=0.00596), while KB-R7943 decreased proliferation in mechanically injured cells by 46 ± 9% (p=0.01991) (**Fig. 2.5B**). The effects of TTX and KB-R7943 on attenuation of injury- induced proliferation were of similar magnitude (p=0.96016), consistent with involvement of VGSC and NCX activities along a common pathway. These findings suggest that attenuation of wound closure by TTX and KB-R7943 is due to combined effects on both migration and proliferation.

2.3.5 $[Ca^{2+}]_i$ is necessary for astrocyte response to injury

There is an extensive literature regarding a contribution of $[Ca^{2+}]_i$ fluxes for cell migration (Schwab et al. 2012) and proliferation (Berridge 1995) in numerous cell types, including astrocytes (Parnis et al. 2013; Stanimirovic et al. 1995; Wang et al. 2010). Given the similar effects of TTX and KB-R7943 on the response of astrocytes to mechanical injury and the non-additivity of their effects, we considered a common pathway involving changes in $[Ca^{2+}]_i$ due to reverse operation of NCX triggered by increased $[Na^+]_i$ via VGSCs, specifically Nav1.5. To test this hypothesis, we first determined whether astroglial response to mechanical injury was dependent on $[Ca^{2+}]$ levels. An intracellular Ca^{2+} chelator, Oregon-Green 488 BAPTA-AM (OGB), was loaded into astrocytes before a scratch injury was performed. After 24 h, OGB-treated cells exhibited only minimal growth into the scratched area (mean gap width = 395 ± 65 µm, n=4), compared to the t=0 scratched area (mean gap width = 414 ± 12 µm, n=31), thereby demonstrating a requirement for $[Ca^{2+}]_i$ levels in the response of astrocytes to mechanical injury.

2.3.6 Astrocytes display a robust [Ca^{2+}]$_i$ response after injury, which is attenuated by TTX and KB- R7943

Given the effect of TTX and KB-R7943 on the response of astrocytes to scratch injury, and the requirement for [Ca^{2+}]$_i$ levels in astrogliosis, we examined [Ca^{2+}]$_i$ dynamics with the calcium indicator Fura-2 AM in astrocytes after mechanical injury. After scratch injury, there was a robust [Ca^{2+}]$_i$ response that propagated through the syncytium of confluent astrocytes, and slowly resolved after 2-4 min (**Fig. 2.6A**, first panel; **Fig. 2.6B**, red line). To determine whether blockade of sodium channels and reverse NCX altered the injury-induced [Ca^{2+}]$_i$ transient in astrocytes, we treated the cells with TTX and KB-R7943 prior to injury and assessed the [Ca^{2+}]$_i$ response. TTX and KB-R7943 each attenuated the initial [Ca^{2+}]$_i$ increase after injury, particularly within the first 60 s (**Fig. 2.6A-C**). Compared to untreated and scratched control astrocytes (n=7 experiments, 70 cells total), TTX decreased the initial 60 s area under curve (AUC) by 21 ± 5% (n=3 experiments, 30 cells total, p=0.01065), while KB-R7943 decreased the initial 60 s AUC by 20 ± 1% (n=3 experiments, 30 cells total, p=0.01355) (**Fig. 2.6C**). In addition, TTX decreased the peak [Ca^{2+}]$_i$ transient by 16 ± 3% (p=0.00395) and KB-R7943 decreased the peak [Ca^{2+}]$_i$ by 12 ± 3% (p=0.02109) compared to scratched and untreated astrocytes (**Fig. 2.6D**). There were not significant differences between the inhibitory effects of TTX and KB-R7943 on the initial 60 s AUCs or the peak Ca^{2+} transients (p=0.9913 and p=0.6613, respectively), consistent with a common pathway contributing to attenuation of [Ca^{2+}]$_i$ response after injury.

2.3.7 Nav1.5 knockdown attenuates astrocytic [Ca^{2+}]$_i$ response after injury

Considering the inhibitory effect of TTX on injury-induced [Ca^{2+}]$_i$ response in astrocytes and the attenuation of wound closure following Nav1.5 siRNA incubation, we determined whether knockdown of Nav1.5 would yield similar attenuation of Ca^{2+} transients in mechanically injured astrocytes. Quantitative real-time PCR confirmed that Nav1.5 mRNA expression of cells treated with Nav1.5 siRNA was decreased by 68 ± 5% compared to NT siRNA (p=0.00002), indicating successful knockdown of Nav1.5 (**Fig. 2.7E**). Compared to NT siRNA (n=3 experiments, 30 cells total), Nav1.5 siRNA (n=5 experiments, 50 cells total) treatment significantly attenuated the [Ca^{2+}]$_i$ response after injury (**Fig. 2.7A, B**). Specifically, knockdown of Nav1.5 decreased the initial 60 s AUC by 18 ± 2% (p=0.00461, **Fig. 2.7C**) and the peak [Ca^{2+}]$_i$ by 18 ± 3% (p=0.04395, **Fig. 2.7D**) compared to NT siRNA. These inhibitory effects on Ca^{2+} transients following Nav1.5 siRNA treatment are similar to those obtained with TTX treatment (AUC decreased 21 ± 5% and peak [Ca^{2+}]$_i$ decreased 16 ± 3%).

2.4 DISCUSSION

The molecular mechanisms that control astroglial scarring following CNS insult are complex and an area of active investigation. Homeostatic functions of astrocytes by way of Na^+ and Ca^{2+} signaling play important roles in both physiological and pathological states (Parpura and Verkhratsky 2012). Here we show, in an *in vitro* model of mechanical injury to astrocytes, that voltage-gated sodium channel (VGSC) Nav1.5, traditionally viewed as a cardiac sodium channel, contributes to the astrocytic response to the insult via triggering reverse mode of the Na^+/Ca^{2+} exchanger (NCX). Our study provides support for a contribution of VGSCs in the pathway leading to astrogliosis following mechanical injury.

The present study contributes to a large body of work investigating the mechanisms that regulate the glial response to injury, both *in vitro* and *in vivo* (for review, see Sofroniew, 2009), which has led to the identification of several critical molecules, and thus potential targets for the modulation of astrogliosis. For example, signal transducer and activator of transcription 3 (STAT3) regulates astrogliosis after crush spinal cord injury (SCI) by promoting proliferation and elongation of astrocytes along glial scar borders (Herrmann et al. 2008; Wanner et al. 2013). The transcription factor Olig2 has also been identified as an important player in astrogliosis by regulating astrocyte proliferation after cortical contusion injury (Chen et al. 2008), and the transcription factor NF-κB was found to markedly affect astrogliosis in both spinal cord injury and experimental autoimmune encephalitis (EAE) (Brambilla et al. 2005; Brambilla et al. 2009a). The implications of modulation of astrogliosis have been explored by targeting these and other molecules in transgenic and knockout *in vivo* models, and both

beneficial (Herrmann et al. 2008; Wanner et al. 2013) and deleterious (Brambilla

et al. 2005; Brambilla et al. 2009a; Okada et al. 2006) effects have been

identified, indicating the heterogeneity of astrogliosis and the complexity of its

effects.

Voltage-gated sodium channels contribute to regulation of motility,

invasion, and proliferation in numerous cell types (for a review of the non-

canonical functions of VGSCs see Black and Waxman, 2013), including immune

cells such as macrophages (Carrithers et al. 2009), microglia (Black and

Waxman 2012), lymphocytes (Fraser et al. 2008), and dendritic cells (Kis-Toth et

al. 2011). Nav1.6 sodium channels are expressed in association with intracellular

membranes within macrophages and appear to participate in pathways that

regulate motility of these cells by causing shifts of intracellular Na^+ and Ca^{2+},

which affect signaling pathways, linking VGSC activation to effects on the

cytoskeleton (Carrithers et al. 2009). Consistent with a contribution of VGSC

activity to cell motility, blockade of VGSCs with TTX attenuates migration of

microglia (Black and Waxman 2012) and invasiveness of T-lymphocytes, with

Nav1.5 specifically being implicated (Fraser et al. 2008). In addition, expression

of VGSCs in dendritic cells contributes to a depolarized membrane potential that

is necessary for cell migration (Kis-Toth et al. 2011). Additionally, VGSCs and

NCX have been implicated in GABA-induced NG2 cell migration by way of fluxes

in $[Ca^{2+}]_i$ (Tong et al. 2009), and Nav1.5 was shown to be involved in both migration (Wu et al. 2008) and proliferation (Wu et al. 2006) of gastric epithelial cells.

In addition to the importance of VGSCs in cell motility and proliferation, it is becoming increasingly recognized that the expression of VGSCs correlates with invasiveness and metastatic potential in many types of cancer cells including prostate (Fraser et al. 2003), breast (Brackenbury et al. 2007; Gillet et al. 2009), and colon (House et al. 2010). Importantly, SCN5A (encoding Nav1.5) has been identified as a driver of human cancer cell invasion in both breast and colon cancer. Electrophysiological analysis of breast cancer cells uncovered sustained Nav1.5 activity (Gillet et al. 2009), and knockdown of Nav1.5 (Brackenbury et al. 2007; Gillet et al. 2009; House et al. 2010) attenuates invasive behavior of these non-excitable cell types. Voltage-gated sodium channels, and specifically Nav1.5, have also been directly linked to $[Ca^{2+}]_i$ shifts in various non-excitable cell types. Nav1.5 in human macrophages regulates the processing of Mycobacteria via organelle polarization and Ca^{2+} oscillations (Carrithers et al. 2011), and it was recently shown that the gene encoding the pore-forming subunit of Nav1.5 triggers a $[Ca^{2+}]_i$ signal that is essential for the positive selection of $CD4^+$ T cells (Lo et al. 2012).

Our results build upon earlier work which demonstrated upregulated expression of Nav1.5 within scarring astrocytes in multiple sclerosis lesions and in other human brain pathologies (Black et al. 2010) and showed that cultured astrocytes display TTX-resistant sodium currents after mechanical injury-induced gliosis (MacFarlane and Sontheimer 1998). Voltage-gated sodium channel activation leads to increased Na^+ influx, which has the capability to increase $[Ca^{2+}]_i$ via the reverse mode of NCX. Because the reversal potential of NCX in astrocytes is set at levels close to the resting membrane potential (Kirischuk et al. 1997; Reyes et al. 2012), NCX can rapidly switch into reverse mode in response to small $[Na^+]_i$ increases and/or depolarization (Kirischuk et al. 2012; Paluzzi et al. 2007). Simultaneous Ca^{2+} and Na^+ waves have in fact been observed after mechanical and electrical stimulation of cultured astrocytes (Bernardinelli et al. 2004). Furthermore, it has been shown that mechanical strain injury increases intracellular sodium and leads to reversal of NCX in cortical astrocytes (Floyd et al. 2005).

It is widely accepted that cell migration is a Ca^{2+}-dependent process, as many components of the migration apparatus are Ca^{2+}-sensitive, including calcineurin, calpain, and Ca^{2+}/calmodulin-dependent protein kinase, among others (for review, see Schwab et al., 2012). The initiation of cell motility following injury is dependent on an initial wound- induced increase in $[Ca^{2+}]_i$, which induces the transcriptional activity of immediate early genes such as c-fos and c-jun (Tran et al. 1999). These genes have been shown to be important for regulating cell motility in endothelial cells through secondary genes coding molecules involved in cellular migration (Tran et al. 1999). Intriguingly, a recent study identified a signaling cascade that contributes to glial scarring in an *in vitro* mechanical injury model similar to ours. Gao et al. (2013) showed that the $[Ca^{2+}]_i$ increase in astrocytes after injury activates the protein kinase JNK, which phosphorylates transcription factor c-jun to facilitate the binding of AP-1 to the

GFAP gene promoter, which in turn allows GFAP upregulation and subsequent scar formation. It is also evident that Ca^{2+} signaling is crucial to the process of cellular proliferation by activating immediate early genes that activate the cell cycle in resting cells (for review, see Berridge, 1995). Given this literature, we suggest that the attenuation of initial $[Ca^{2+}]_i$ response by TTX and KB-R7943 impacts longer-term scar formation by affecting transcriptional activity of immediate early genes (e.g. via JNK/c-jun/AP-1 signaling cascade), which regulate secondary genes important for cell migration and cell proliferation. In support of this proposed mechanism, we found no significant difference between the effects of TTX treatment for 15 minutes versus 2 hours versus 24 hours, indicating that the time-frame for blockade of VGSCs to affect wound closure is early, which corresponds to the early $[Ca^{2+}]_i$ response. Additionally, treatment with the Ca^{2+} chelator Oregon-Green 488 BAPTA-AM (OGB) at the time of cellular injury inhibited the astrocyte response to scratch injury, again implicating the initial $[Ca^{2+}]_i$ increase as a regulator of astrocyte wound closure.

Since astrocytes are highly coupled via gap junctions, supporting conduction of Na^+, Ca^{2+}, and other molecules (Parpura and Verkhratsky 2012; Spray et al. 2006) to adjacent astrocytes (Konietzko and Müller 1994), we propose that mechanical injury depolarizes injured cells along the edge of the scratch, and that this depolarization spreads via gap junctions to neighboring cells, activating Nav1.5 and further increasing $[Na^+]_i$ and/or depolarization. The increased intracellular Na^+ gradient would be expected to drive NCX in reverse, or Ca^{2+} importing, mode, thereby increasing $[Ca^{2+}]_i$, and leading to wound closure by Ca^{2+}-dependent migration and proliferation mechanisms, including activation

of gene transcription as detailed in Gao et al. (2013) (**Fig. 2.8**).

Reactive astrogliosis is an important aspect of CNS pathologies and

although milder forms of astrogliosis may have beneficial effects to the healing of

the CNS, it is possible that attenuating the more severe glial scar formation could

be beneficial in disease states such as multiple sclerosis, traumatic brain injury

(TBI), and spinal cord injury (SCI). Previous studies on *in vivo* models of multiple

sclerosis have shown improved clinical status and reduction of axonal loss

following treatment with a variety of VGSC blockers including phenytoin (Black et

al. 2007), lamotrigine (Bechtold et al. 2006), carbamazepine (Black et al. 2007),

safinamide, and flecainide (Morsali et al. 2013). Interestingly, flecainide, which is

a Class Ic cardiac anti-arrhythmic, has strong state-dependent effects on Nav1.5

(Ramos and O'Leary 2004). Additionally, phenytoin protects spinal cord axons,

reduces gray and white matter destruction surrounding the lesion, and improves

functional recovery after contusion-induced SCI (Hains et al. 2004) and

phenytoin, riluzole, and mexilitine were all shown to improve outcome after spinal

cord injury in rodents (Ates et al. 2007). Whether an attenuation of astrogliosis

due to sodium channel blockade contributes to the improved outcomes is not

clear.

In summary, our observations in astrocytes *in vitro* demonstrate a

molecular mechanism involving VGSC and NCX that contributes to the glial

response to injury. Specifically, our results show that reverse Na^+/Ca^{2+} exchange, triggered by Nav1.5 channels, plays an important role in pathways regulating the

response of astrocytes to injury.

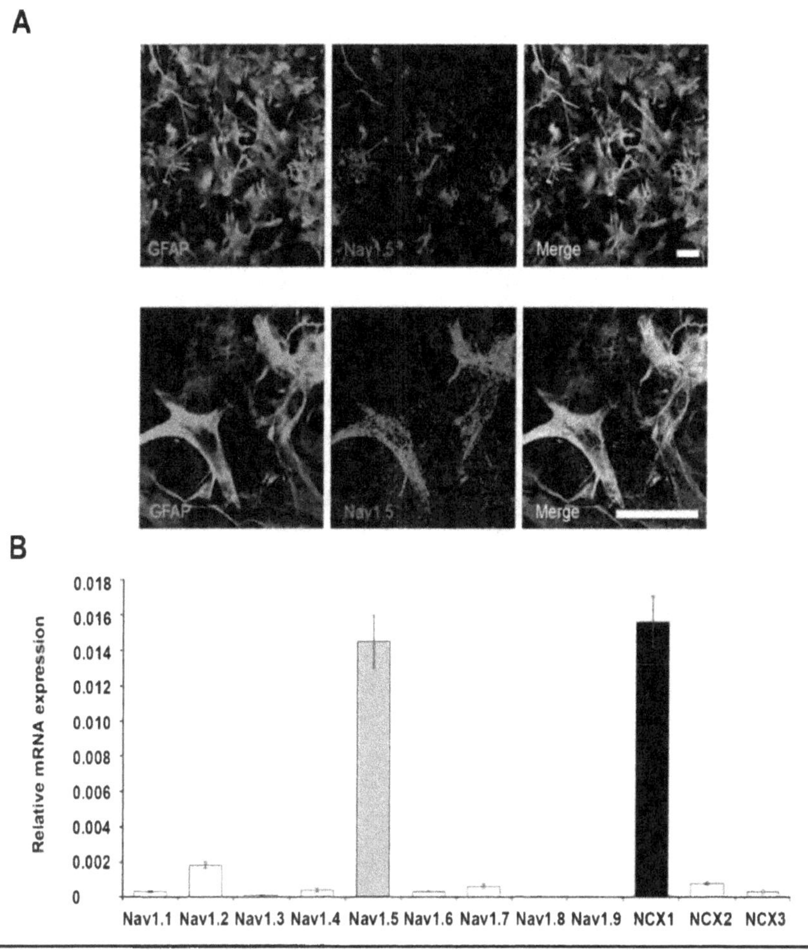

Figure 2.1 – Nav1.5 and NCX1 expression in astrocytes. **(A)** GFAP-positive cultured rat cortical astrocytes (green) exhibit prominent Nav1.5 immunolabeling (red), observed at low magnification (top panel) and at increased magnification (bottom panel). Merged images of GFAP and Nav1.5 are yellow. Scale bars, 25 μm. **(B)** RT-PCR showing relative mRNA expression of VGSCs and NCX. Nav1.5 is the predominant VGSC subtype expressed in cultured rat cortical astrocytes and the NCX1 isoform is also robustly expressed. *Data in 2.1B generated by OA Samad.*

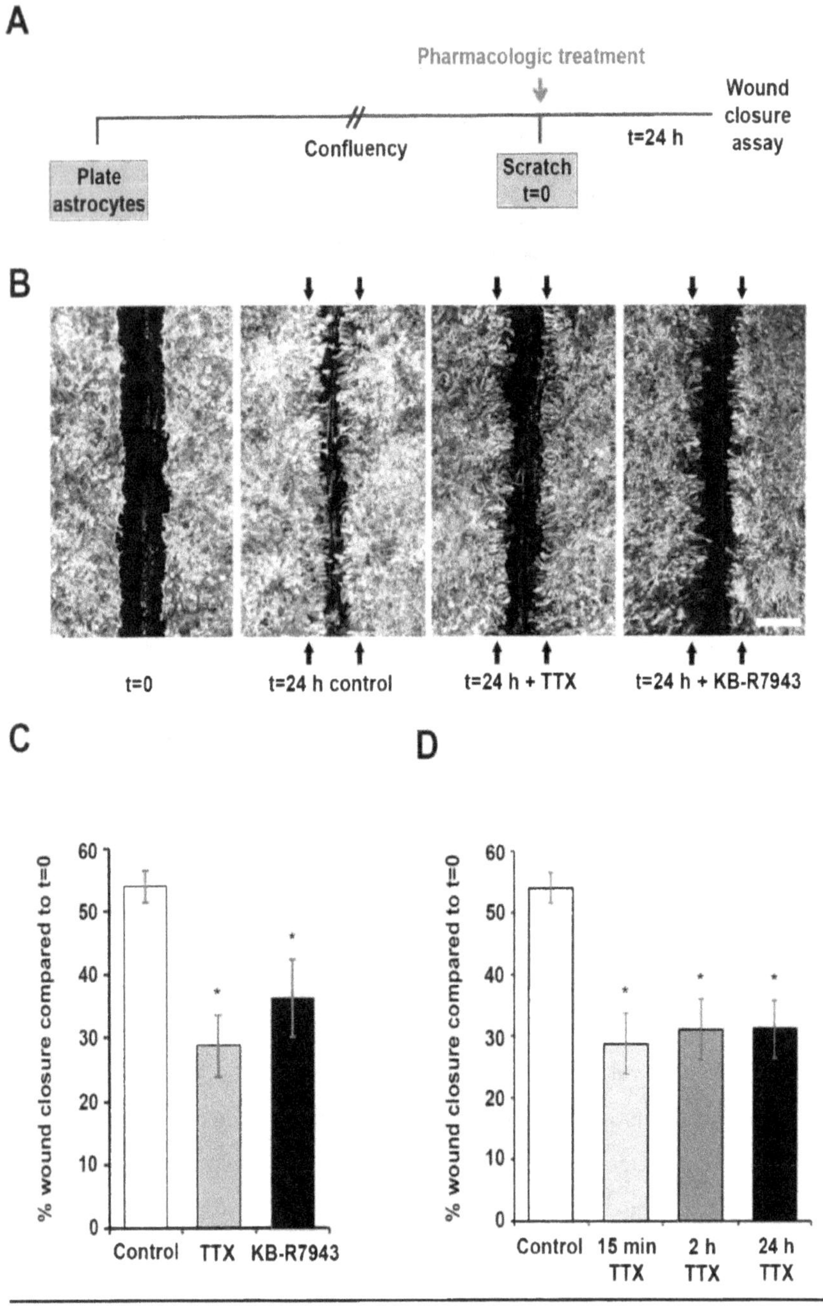

A
Pharmacologic treatment
Wound closure assay
Confluency
t=24 h
Plate astrocytes
Scratch t=0

B
t=0
t=24 h control
t=24 h + TTX
t=24 h + KB-R7943

C
% wound closure compared to t=0
Control
TTX
KB-R7943

D
% wound closure compared to t=0
Control
15 min TTX
2 h TTX
24 h TTX

Figure 2.2 – Astrocyte response to mechanical injury is inhibited by TTX and KB-R7943. (A) Schematic of experimental design. Astrocytes were plated and allowed to grow until confluent, at which point they were treated with either TTX or KB-R7943 and scratched. After 24 h, wound closure was analyzed and compared to initial wound size. **(B, C)** Astrocytes grew together following scratch injury, resulting in 54 ± 3% (n=29) closure of the wound compared to the average original wound size (represented by black arrows) after a 24 h period. TTX treatment attenuated closure of the scratch wound to 28 ± 5% (n=15) of the initial wound size at t=24 h. Similarly, KB-R7943 inhibited wound closure, with 36 ± 6% regrowth (n=6) of the initial scratch size. **(D)** TTX, applied for 15 min or 2 h after scratch, was compared to TTX applied for the full 24 h period prior to assessment at 24 h. After 24 h, there were significant differences between the degree of wound closure for untreated scratched controls (54 ± 5%, n=7) and for TTX treatment for 15 min (31 ± 5%, n=5), 2 h (31 ± 5%, n=6), and 24 h (30 ± 8%, n=5). There was no significant difference between the effects of TTX for 15 min, 2 h, and 24 h. Scale bar, 400 μm. *p<0.05.

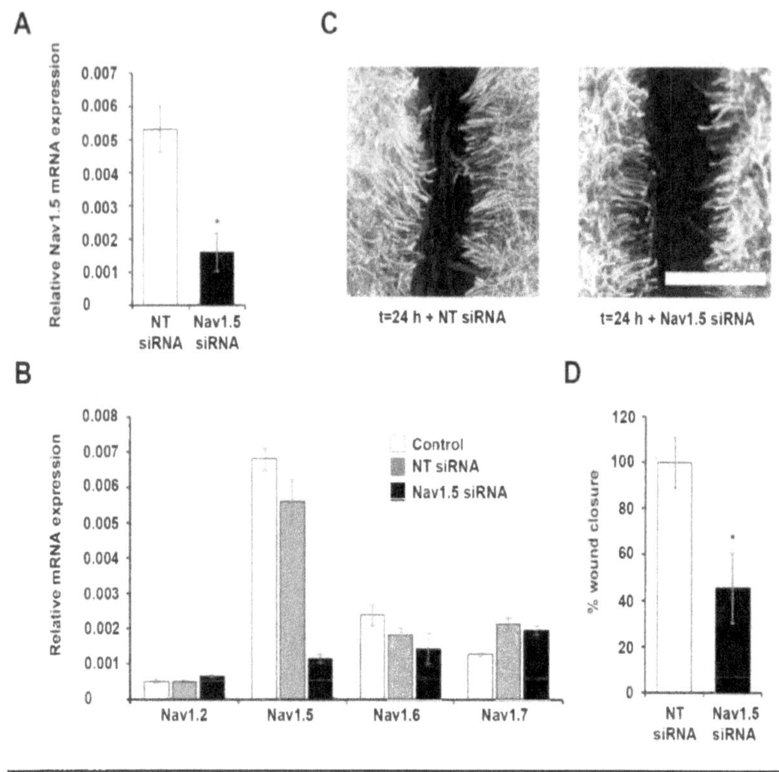

Figure 2.3 – Astrocyte response to injury is inhibited by Nav1.5 mRNA knockdown. (A) Quantitative real-time PCR was performed and showed that Nav1.5 mRNA expression of cells treated with Nav1.5 siRNA was decreased by 70 ± 11% compared to NT siRNA, indicating successful knockdown of Nav1.5. **(B)** Specificity of the Nav1.5 siRNA cocktail on Nav1.5 mRNA expression was confirmed with real-time PCR analysis. Compared to control (white columns), minimal effects of NT siRNA (gray columns) or Nav1.5 siRNA (black columns) on the expression of Nav1.2, Nav1.6, and Nav1.7 mRNA were observed. **(C, D)** Twenty-four hours after the scratch injury, exposure to Nav1.5 siRNA (n=6) reduced the amount of wound closure to 45 ± 15% compared to NT siRNA (n=6). Scale bar, 400 µm. *p<0.05.

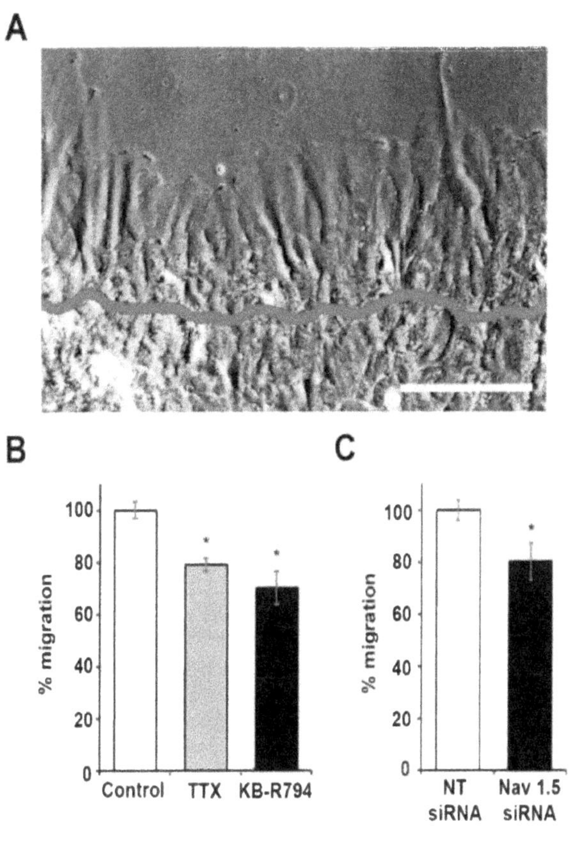

Figure 2.4 – Astrocyte response to injury involves migration which is attenuated by TTX, KB-R7943, and Nav1.5 mRNA knockdown. (A) After a scrape-induced injury (original site of injury marked by red line), astrocytic processes are seen extending. After 24 h, cell processes had migrated 136 ± 20 µm from the site of injury in control conditions. Scale bar, 150 µm. (B) Compared to untreated cells (n=9), TTX decreased migration by 21 ± 3% (n=3) and KB-R7943 decreased migration by 30 ± 6% (n=5). (C) Compared to treated with NT siRNA (n=4), astrocytes treated with Nav1.5 siRNA exhibited a 20 ± 7% decrease in migration (n=3). *p<0.05.

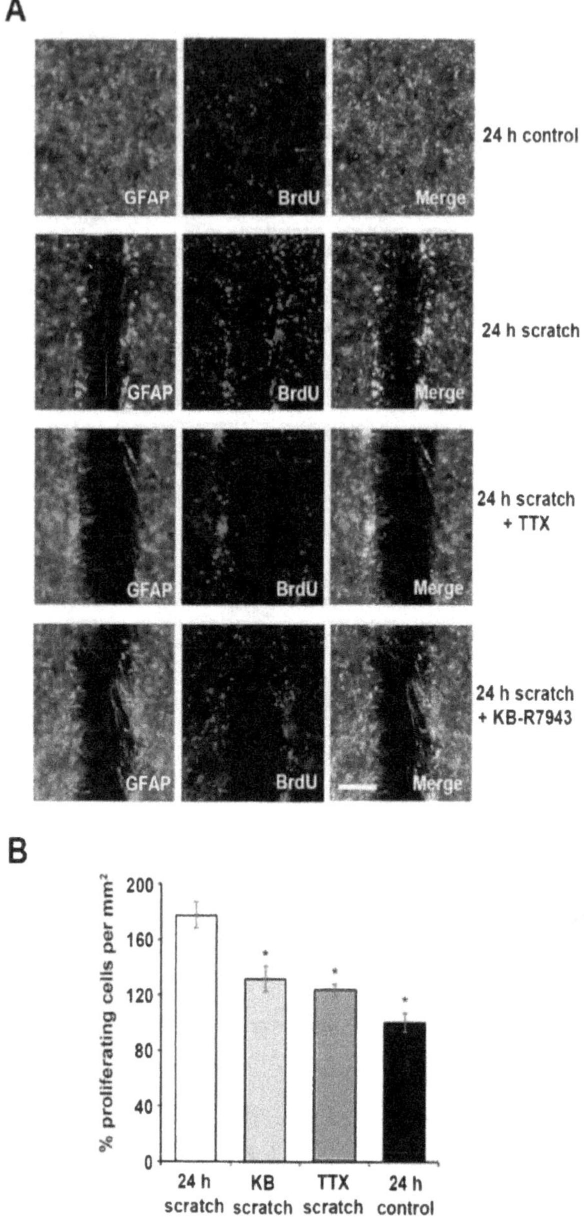

A
GFAP
BrdU
Merge
24 h control
GFAP
BrdU
Merge
24 h scratch
GFAP
BrdU
Merge
24 h scratch
+ TTX
GFAP
BrdU
Merge
24 h scratch
+ KB-R7943
B
% proliferating cells per mm²
200
160
120
80
40
0
24 h
scratch
KB
scratch
TTX
scratch
24 h
control

Figure 2.5 – Astrocyte response to injury involves proliferation which is attenuated by TTX and KB-R7943. (A) GFAP-positive cultured rat cortical astrocytes (green) exhibit BrdU immunolabeling (red), seen in resting cells (top row) and scratched cells (second row). There is an increase in BrdU-positive cells along the edge of a scratch, which is attenuated with TTX and KB-R7943 treatment (third and fourth rows, respectively). Scale bar 200 μm. **(B)** After 24 h, there was a significant 77 ± 9% increase in proliferation amongst cells along the edge of a wound (n=7) compared to cells in unscratched cultures (n=8), as measured by BrdU staining. Compared to untreated cells, TTX decreased proliferation by 54 ± 4%, while KB-R7943 decreased proliferation by 46 ± 9%. *p<0.05; n.s., not significant.

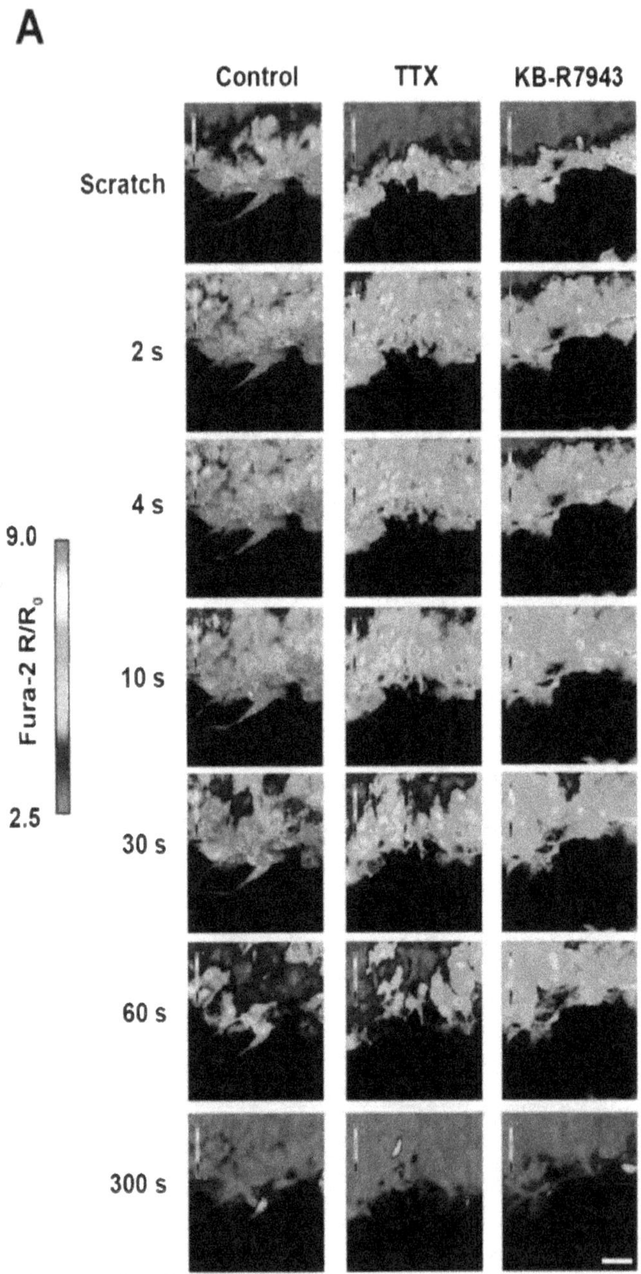
A
Control
TTX
KB-R7943
Scratch
2 s
4 s
10 s
30 s
60 s
300 s
9.0
Fura-2 R/R0
2.5

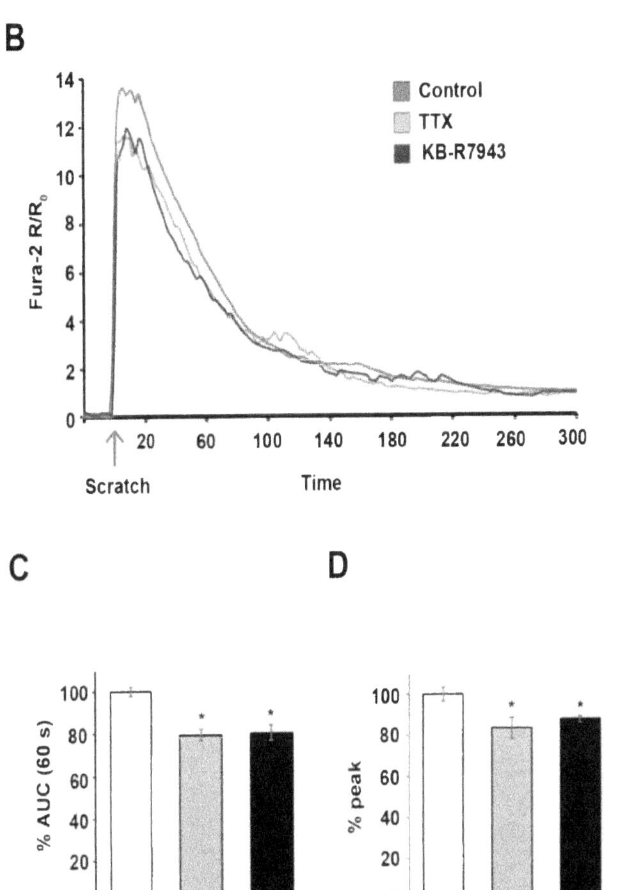

B
14
12
10
8
6
4
2
0
Fura-2 R/R₀
Control
TTX
KB-R7943
20
60
100
140
180
220
260
300
Scratch
Time
C
100
80
60
40
20
0
% AUC (60 s)
*
*
Control
TTX
KB-R7943
D
100
80
60
40
20
0
% peak
*
*
Control
TTX
KB-R7943

Figure 2.6 – Astrocytes display robust [Ca^{2+}]$_i$ response after mechanical injury that is attenuated by TTX and KB-R7943. (A) After a scratch injury, there was a robust [Ca^{2+}]$_i$ response, which was propagated through the syncytium of confluent astrocytes and slowly resolved after 2-4 min. Application of TTX and KB- R7943 attenuated this [Ca^{2+}]$_i$ response (second and third columns, respectively). Color scale represents the ratio of fluorescent signals induced by 340 and 380 nm excitation in cells loaded with Fura-2 AM. Scale bar, 50 µm. **(B)** TTX and KB-R7943 both attenuated the initial [Ca^{2+}]$_i$ increase after injury, particularly within the first 60 s. **(C)** Compared to untreated scratched astrocytes (n=7 experiments, 70 cells total), TTX decreased the 60 s AUC by 21 ± 5% (n=3 experiments, 30 cells total), while KB-R7943 decreased the 60 s AUC by 20 ± 1% (n=3 experiments, 30 cells total). **(D)** TTX decreased the peak [Ca^{2+}]$_i$ by 16 ± 3%, while KB-R7943 decreased the peak [Ca^{2+}]$_i$ by 12 ± 3%. All data was taken from cells within the first 50 µm (3-4 cells deep) from the scratch. *p<0.05; n.s., not significant.

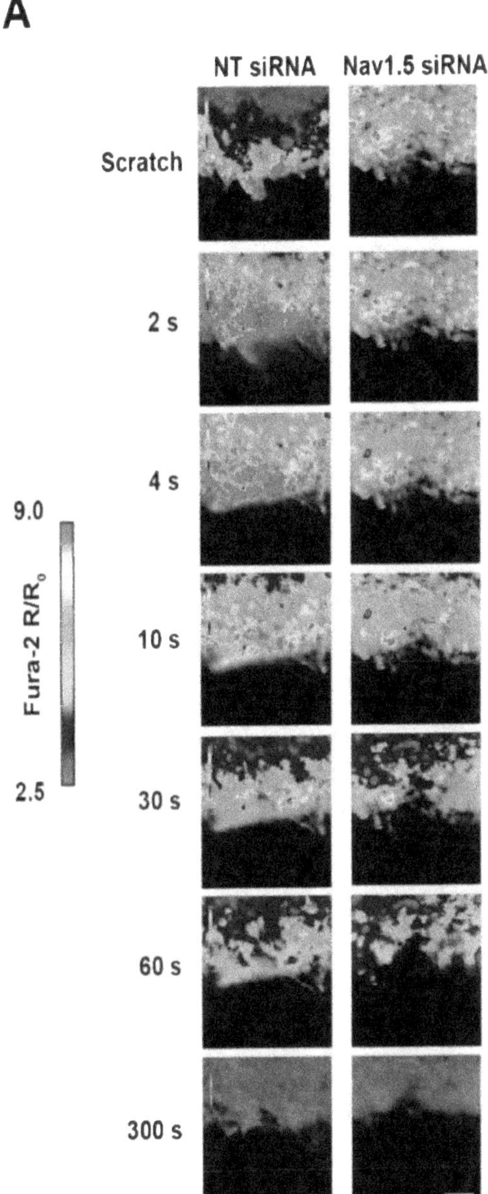

A
NT siRNA
Nav1.5 siRNA
Scratch
2 s
4 s
10 s
30 s
60 s
300 s
9.0
Fura-2 R/R₀
2.5

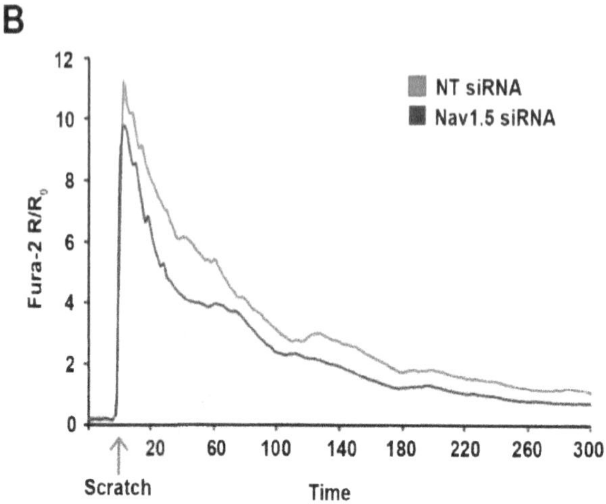

B
12
10
8
6
4
2
0
Fura-2 R/R₀
NT siRNA
Nav1.5 siRNA
20
60
100
140
180
220
260
300
Scratch
Time

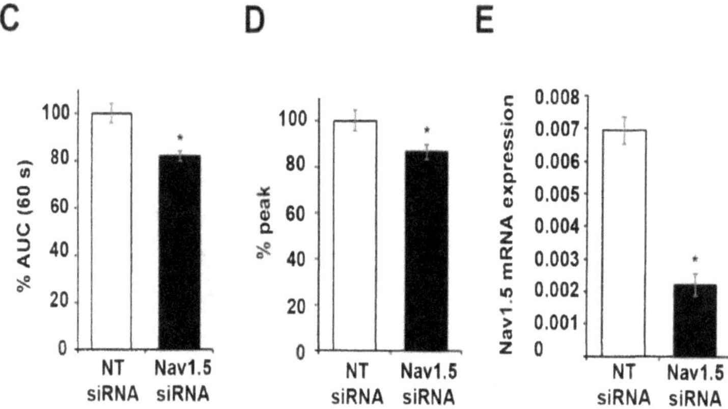

C
100
80
60
40
20
0
% AUC (60 s)
*
NT siRNA
Nav1.5 siRNA
D
100
80
60
40
20
0
% peak
*
NT siRNA
Nav1.5 siRNA
E
0.008
0.007
0.006
0.005
0.004
0.003
0.002
0.001
0
Nav1.5 mRNA expression
*
NT siRNA
Nav1.5 siRNA

Figure 2.7 – Nav1.5 mRNA knockdown attenuates astrocytic $[Ca^{2+}]_i$ response after injury. **(A)** After scratch, there was a robust $[Ca^{2+}]_i$ response in cells treated with NT siRNA, which was propagated through the syncytium of astrocytes and slowly resolved after 2-4 min (first column). Knockdown with Nav1.5 siRNA attenuated the $[Ca^{2+}]_i$ response (second column) compared to NT siRNA. Color scale represents the ratio of fluorescent signals induced by 340 and 380 nm excitation in cells loaded with Fura-2 AM. Scale bar 50 μm. **(B)** Nav1.5 siRNA attenuated the initial $[Ca^{2+}]_i$ increase after injury, particularly within the first 60 s. **(C)** Compared to NT siRNA control (n=5 experiments, 50 cells total), Nav1.5 siRNA treatment (n=3 experiments, 30 cells total) decreased the 60 s AUC by 18 ± 2%, and **(D)** decreased the peak $[Ca^{2+}]_i$ by 18 ± 3%. **(E)** Quantitative real-time PCR confirmed that Nav1.5 mRNA expression of cells treated with Nav1.5 siRNA was decreased by 68 ± 5% compared to NT siRNA, indicating successful knockdown of Nav1.5. All data was taken from cells within the first 50 μm (3-4 cells deep) from the scratch. *p<0.05.

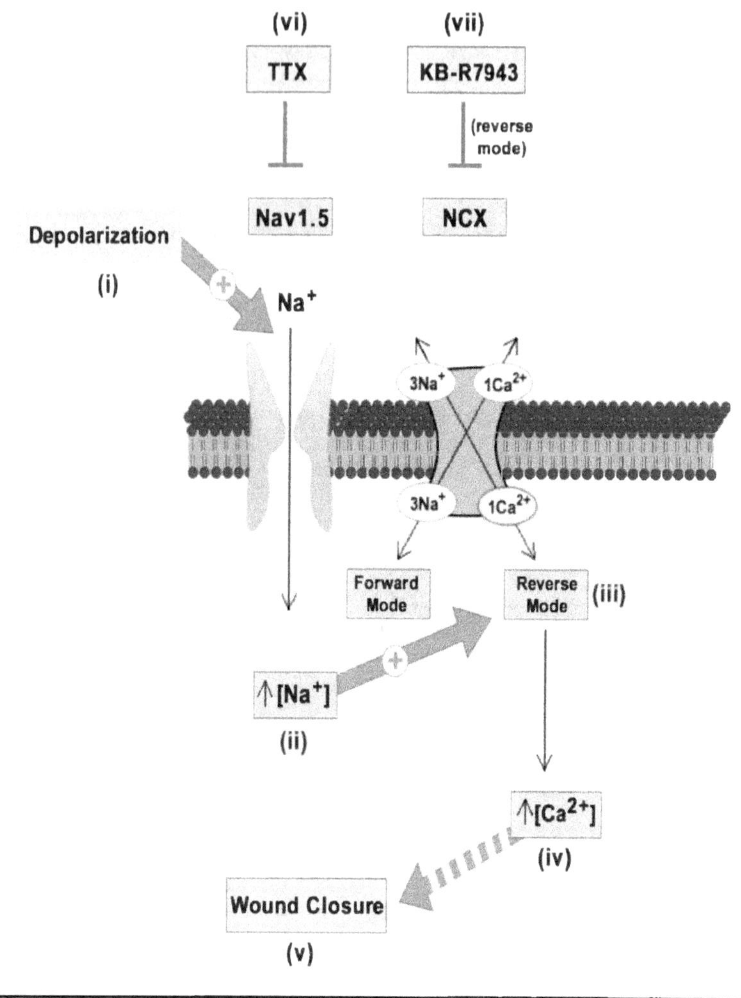

Figure 2.8 Schematic of contribution of Nav1.5 and NCX to astrocyte response following scratch injury. Injury-induced depolarization (i) activates Nav1.5, which causes an increased [Na$^+$]$_i$ and further depolarization (ii). Increased [Na$^+$]$_i$ activates the reverse operation of NCX (Ca^{2+}-importing mode) (iii), which causes increased [Ca^{2+}]$_i$ (iv) that likely acts through multiple pathways (including migration and proliferation) to affect astroglial wound closure (v). TTX (vi) and KB-R7943 (vii) inhibit Nav1.5 and NCX, respectively, thereby attenuating closure of the wound.

CHAPTER 3: DYNAMICS OF NAV1.5 EXPRESSION IN ASTROCYTES IN MOUSE MODELS OF MULTIPLE SCLEROSIS

This chapter contains a modified version of material that appeared in the author's publication: Pappalardo LW, Liu SL, Black JA, Waxman SG (2014). Dynamics of sodium channel Nav1.5 expression in astrocytes in mouse models of multiple sclerosis. Neuroreport 25:1208-1215.

3.1   INTRODUCTION

Though astrocytes have traditionally been considered to be electrically unexcitable, studies since the 1990s have demonstrated that these cells express voltage-gated sodium channels (VGSCs) (Sontheimer et al. 1996), including the isotype Nav1.5 (Black et al. 1998; Pappalardo et al. 2014b). These studies suggest that expression of VGSCs in rodent astrocytes is a dynamic process, changing with response to injury, age, and exposure to the extracellular milieu (MacFarlane and Sontheimer 1998; Sontheimer et al. 1991; Thio and Sontheimer 1993). Notably, Black et al. demonstrated the presence of Nav1.5 in human scarring astrocytes *in situ* within acute and chronic multiple sclerosis (MS) lesions, and surrounding cerebrovascular accidents and central nervous system (CNS) tumors, suggesting a commonality of upregulated astrocytic Nav1.5 following CNS tissue injury (Black et al. 2010).

Despite the well-characterized expression of VGSCs in both rodent and human astrocytes, the functional role of these VGSCs has remained elusive. Astrocytes serve multiple functions in the CNS, including ionic homeostasis and neuronal support. Sontheimer et al. suggested that VGSCs provide a route for $[Na^+]_i$ influx necessary for Na^+/K^+-ATPase function within astrocytes and thus participate in K^+ homeostasis in the CNS (Sontheimer et al. 1994). Astrocytes are also important contributors to the response of the CNS to neuroinflammatory pathologies, including MS. One such response is reactive astrogliosis, which can exhibit both beneficial and detrimental effects to the CNS (Sofroniew 2009). Severe forms of astrogliosis involve formation of a scar that is long-lasting and can inhibit the regeneration of injured neurons (Silver and Miller 2004). Recent work has shown that Nav1.5 plays an important role in an *in vitro* model of glial injury by triggering reverse mode operation of the Na^+-Ca^{2+} exchanger (NCX) (Pappalardo et al. 2014b). These results suggest that Nav1.5 and NCX are potential targets for modulation of astrogliosis after injury via their effect on $[Ca^{2+}]_i$.

Given the dynamic expression of VGSCs in rodent astrocytes (MacFarlane and Sontheimer 1998; Sontheimer et al. 1991; Thio and Sontheimer 1993), the upregulation of Nav1.5 in human scarring astrocytes (Black et al. 2010), and the functional role of Nav1.5 in glial scar formation *in vitro* (Pappalardo et al. 2014b), we examined the temporal dynamics of Nav1.5 expression in scarring astrocytes in neuroinflammatory pathologies, with respect to disease severity and periods of relapse/remission. Here, we investigate the expression of astrocytic Nav1.5 in two mouse models of MS, monophasic experimental autoimmune encephalomyelitis (EAE) and chronic-relapsing EAE (CR EAE). We show that Nav1.5 upregulation correlates to disease severity and that Nav1.5 expression in astrocytes is modulated in parallel with periods of

disease and remission.

3.2   MATERIALS AND METHODS

3.2.1 Induction of EAE

Experiments were carried out in accordance with NIH guidelines for the care and use of laboratory animals; all animal protocols were approved by the IACUC of VA Connecticut Healthcare System, West Haven, CT. C57BL/6 (Harlan, Indianapolis, IN) and Biozzi (Harlan Sera-Lab Ltd, Loughborough, UK) mice 6–10 weeks of age were injected subcutaneously in the flank with 200 µl of an emulsion of 300 µg of rat myelin-oligodendrocyte glycoprotein (MOG) 35–55 peptide (W. M. Keck Biotechnology Resource Center, Yale University) in incomplete Freund's adjuvant (IFA; Sigma, St Louis, MO) supplemented with 500 µg of Mycobacterium tuberculosis H37Ra (Difco, Detroit, MI), as described previously (Black et al. 2006). The MOG injection, with mycobacterium supplemented IFA, was repeated in the contralateral flank 1 week later. The mice also received an injection of 250 ng pertussis toxin (Sigma) in 200 µl phosphate-buffered saline (PBS) intraperitoneally (i.p.) immediately after the first immunization with MOG and then again 48 h later. In agreement with previous descriptions, the C57BL/6 mice developed a monophasic clinical course, while the Biozzi mice exhibited a chronic-relapsing (CR) clinical phenotype (Croxford and Miyake 2016). Control animals received the same injections, with the omission of MOG. A total of 18 C57BL/6 and 20 Biozzi mice were injected.

3.2.2 Clinical assessment

Immunized mice were observed daily and scored on a 0 to 5 clinical scale with increasing clinical score reflecting clinical worsening as follows: 1—flaccid tail; 2—abnormal righting reflex and/or abnormal gait in the absence of weakness; 3—partial hindlimb paralysis; 4—complete hindlimb paralysis; 5—moribund (Matthaei et al. 1989). We applied the scale in 0.5 increments. To characterize the clinical course of CR EAE, the initial episode was defined as a clinical score of ≥ 2.0 for two or more consecutive days. Subsequent relapses were identified by clinical scoring increases of at least 1.0 and defined remissions were identified by clinical scoring decreases of at least 1.0. To estimate overall clinical burden of disease in CR EAE, mean clinical score was determined by averaging clinical scores for all sick days of each animal.

3.2.3 Tissue collection

Mice were sacrificed at varying relapse-remission phases and lengths of disease (range 9-59 days) from date of induction of EAE. Mice were anesthetized with ketamine/xylazine (80/5 mg/kg i.p.) and perfused through the heart with phosphate-buffered saline (PBS) and then with 4% paraformaldehyde in 0.14 M Sorensen's phosphate buffer. Spinal cords and brains were carefully excised, cryoprotected with 30% sucrose in PBS and frozen.

3.2.4 Immunocytochemistry

Twelve µm transverse sections of L1-L2 spinal cords and sagittal sections

of the cortices (bregma 0-1 mm, M2) were cut and incubated with primary

antibodies [mouse anti-glial fibrillary acidic protein (GFAP), 1:1000, Covance,

Princeton, NJ, catalog #SMI-22R; rabbit anti-Nav1.5, 1:100, Alomone,

Jerusalem, Israel, catalog #ASC-013] overnight at 4° C on a rotating shaker.

Sections were rinsed 3 times with phosphate-buffered saline (PBS) and

incubated with secondary antibodies [donkey anti-mouse immunoglobulin G-

Alexa Fluor 488, 1:1000, Invitrogen, Grand Island, NY, cat #P-11065; donkey

anti-rabbit immunoglobulin G Cy3, 1:500, Jackson, West Grove, PA, cat #711-

165-152] overnight. Slides were rinsed with PBS and coverslips were mounted

with Aqua Poly mount (Polysciences, Warrington, PA). Control experiments were

performed with the omission of the primary antibodies and only background

labeling was observed.

3.2.5 Data Acquisition and analysis

Multiple images of control, C57BL/6, and Biozzi tissues were obtained with

a Nikon C1*si* confocal microscope (Nikon USA, Melville, NY) operating under

identical gain settings with frame lambda (sequential) mode and saturation

indicator activated to prevent possible bleed-through between channels. For

quantitative analysis of Nav1.5, NIS Elements software was utilized. For C57BL/6

animals (monophasic EAE), high magnification images of astrocytes in the

anterolateral white matter in the L1-L2 region of the spinal cord were selected for analysis. Regions of interest for mean RGB intensity analysis were created by manually outlining individual astrocytes based on GFAP staining. Multiple high magnification images for each animal were taken, quantified, and averaged. For description of astrocytic expression of Nav1.5 in the motor cortex, high magnification images of astrocytes in the parasagittal motor cortex (bregma 0-1 mm, M2) were obtained.

For Biozzi animals (CR EAE), low magnification images of the L1-L2 region of the spinal cord were analyzed. To quantify astrocytic Nav1.5 levels, thresholds were set at the same value for all images by creating a binary layer based on visible GFAP staining in control tissues. Subsequently, regions of interest were manually defined in anterolateral white matter and the RGB mean intensity of the region of interest was extracted within the binary layer. Multiple low magnification images for each animal were taken, quantified, and averaged. One of the twenty Biozzi EAE animals was excluded secondary to poor tissue quality due to severity of disease. Images were composed and processed to enhance contrast in the figures in Adobe Photoshop, with identical settings for the different conditions.

3.2.6 Statistical methods

Clinical scores for C57/B6 animals (monophasic EAE) were represented by clinical score on the day of euthanasia. Clinical scores for Biozzi animals (CR EAE) were computed by averaging the clinical scores for each day to estimate mean overall disease severity. To assess correlation between Nav1.5

immunolabeling and animal clinical status, correlation coefficients (Spearman for normally distributed data; Pearson for nonparametric data) and two-tailed p-values were calculated with GraphPad Prism (GraphPad Software, La Jolla, CA). Data were normalized to percent fluorescence compared to control animals.

3.3   RESULTS

Astrocytes in control human brain do not display sodium channel Nav1.5 immunolabeling above background levels but exhibit robust Nav1.5 immunofluorescence within acute and chronic multiple sclerosis (MS) lesions. To examine the temporal pattern of Nav1.5 expression in astrocytes and the relationship of the degree of Nav1.5 expression to disease severity in a murine model of MS, we examined tissue from mice with acute monophasic and chronic-relapsing experimental autoimmune encephalomyelitis (EAE).

3.3.1   Spinal cord and motor cortex astrocytes in mice with monophasic EAE exhibit upregulated Nav1.5 expression

Astrocytes within the spinal cord anterolateral white matter of control C57BL/6 mice did not display Nav1.5 immunolabeling above background levels (**Fig. 3.1A**). In contrast, the progression of clinical severity in C57BL/6 mice with monophasic EAE was associated with increasing levels of Nav1.5 immunofluorescence (**Fig. 3.1B**). Nav1.5 labeling was detectable at low levels above background in astrocytes from mice with EAE with a clinical score of 2.5 (abnormal righting reflex/mild weakness in hindlimbs), while robust Nav1.5 reactivity was generally exhibited by astrocytes in mice with clinical scores greater than 4.0 (complete hindlimb paralysis).

As shown in **Fig. 3.1B**, quantification of the Nav1.5 immunofluorescence in astrocytes within spinal cord anterolateral white matter of mice with monophasic EAE yielded a positive correlation between mean astrocytic Nav1.5

signal and clinical score (R=0.7131, p=0.009, n=18), consistent with increased expression of Nav1.5 within astrocytes as mice with monophasic EAE exhibited increasing disease severity.

The enhanced Nav1.5 immunofluorescence in astrocytes with increasing clinical score was also manifest in astrocytes within different regions of the CNS. For example, astrocytes within motor cortex of mice with monophasic EAE exhibited increased Nav1.5 immunolabeling with increasing disease severity, as observed in **Fig. 3.1C**.

3.3.2 Spinal cord astrocytes in mice with chronic-relapsing EAE display upregulated Nav1.5 expression

To assess the disease severity of Biozzi mice with chronic-relapsing EAE (CR EAE), totals of the clinical score at each day following the onset of the disease (clinical score >1.0) to euthanasia were calculated and then divided by the number of days in the disease state, to yield a mean clinical score, reflective of overall disease burden. As exemplified in **Fig. 3.2A**, astrocytes within spinal cord anterolateral white matter exhibited enhanced Nav1.5 immunofluorescence with increasing mean clinical score. Quantification of the mean astrocytic Nav1.5 signal intensity yielded a positive correlation (R=0.7541, p=0.0002, n=19) with increasing mean clinical score (**Fig. 3.2B**).

3.3.3 Astrocytic Nav1.5 is attenuated during periods of remission in chronic-relapsing EAE

We also determined whether the level of Nav1.5 immunolabeling in astrocytes in Biozzi mice with chronic-relapsing EAE was altered in remitting and relapsing phases of the disease. As shown in **Fig. 3.3A**, MOG inoculation of Biozzi mice induced a relapsing-remitting form of EAE, with mean clinical scores of ~2.5 in the first episode and first relapse and ~1.8 and ~2.0 in the first and second remissions, respectively. Astrocytes within spinal cord anterolateral white matter displayed Nav1.5 immunofluorescent signals that paralleled the relapsing-remitting clinical course (**Fig. 3.3B**). Quantification of Nav1.5 immunofluorescence in astrocytes in the chronic-relapsing phases is provided in **Fig. 3.3C** and was consistent with an upregulation of Nav1.5 in astrocytes in the first episode that was attenuated in the 1st remission, further upregulated in the 1st episode, and again attenuated in the 2nd remission.

3.4　DISCUSSION

Previous studies have shown that rodent astrocytes express voltage-gated sodium channels (VGSCs) (for review see Sontheimer et al. 1996), including Nav1.5 sodium channels (Black et al. 1998; Pappalardo et al. 2014b). Black et al. (1998) demonstrated Nav1.5 mRNA and protein in rodent astrocytes *in vitro* and *in situ* and Black et al. (2010) showed upregulated expression of Nav1.5 in astrocytes associated with acute and chronic multiple sclerosis (MS) lesions, new and old stroke lesions, and central nervous system (CNS) tumors, including gliomas and a metastatic carcinoma (Black et al. 1998; Black et al. 2010). However, the temporal sequence of Nav1.5 expression in activated astrocytes has yet to be established. Here, we examine the expression of astrocytic Nav1.5 in different phases of monophasic and chronic-relapsing (CR) EAE models of MS. We show that Nav1.5 upregulation in astrocytes correlates with disease severity of the mice, as indicated by clinical score. The low level of Nav1.5 expression in astrocytes of control animals suggests that Nav1.5 upregulation is part of the biological response of astrocytes to CNS insult.

The expression of Nav1.5, which is tetrodotoxin-resistant (TTX-R) (Rogart et al. 1989) in astrocytes appears to be a dynamic process, changing with regard to age of the animal and culture conditions, exposure to extracellular factors, and response to injury (MacFarlane and Sontheimer 1998; Pappalardo et al. 2014b; Sontheimer et al. 1991; Thio and Sontheimer 1993). MacFarlane and Sontheimer described a shift from TTX-sensitive (TTX-S) sodium currents to TTX-R sodium currents with properties ascribed to Nav1.5 in rodent astrocytes in an *in vitro* model of glial injury (MacFarlane and Sontheimer 1998). Our finding that Nav1.5 expression in astrocytes is modulated in parallel with clinical course of the animal is consistent with the notion that Nav1.5 is regulated temporally in astrocytes in response to neuroinflammation.

Astrocytes perform multiple functions in the CNS, and the functional roles of VGSCs in astrocytes is incompletely understood, although studies have provided certain insight (for review of noncanonical roles of VGSCs in astrocytes and other non-excitable cell types, see Black and Waxman, 2013). It has been shown that VGSCs in astrocytes can be localized to the plasma membrane, where they are capable of producing sodium currents (Barres et al. 1989). A standing Na^+ influx in astrocytes is critical for Na^+/K^+-ATPase activity and Sontheimer et al. proposed that VGSCs channels provide a pathway for Na^+ to enter the cell to maintain $[Na^+]_i$ at levels necessary for Na^+/K^+-ATPase activity (Sontheimer et al. 1994). This action, in turn, supports the regulation of ionic homeostasis in the CNS, with regards to K^+ fluxes. Inglese et al. demonstrated through ^{23}Na MRI that sodium concentrations are elevated in acute and chronic MS lesions when compared to normal appearing white matter (NAWM) (Inglese et al. 2010), which may be related to the suggestion of Black et al. (2010) that upregulation of Nav1.5 may provide a compensatory mechanism to support ionic homeostasis mediated by Na^+/K^+-ATPase activity in areas of CNS damage (Black et al. 2010).

In addition to other functions in the CNS, astrocytes are prominent participants in the response to inflammatory insults through the process of

reactive astrogliosis, which occurs following injury in many CNS pathologies,
including MS. Although activated astrocytes can exert beneficial and detrimental
actions following CNS injury (Sofroniew 2009), recent work has linked pro-
inflammatory effects of activated astrocytes as critical contributors to the
inflammatory response in EAE (Brambilla et al. 2014). In addition, severe forms
of astrogliosis are associated with the formation of a glial scar, which is often
persistent and can impede neuronal regeneration after injury (Silver and Miller
2004).

Accumulating evidence indicates a role of $[Na^+]_i$ transients in contributing
to astroglial excitability and cellular homeostasis, with a prominent mechanism
involving the linkage of transmembrane movements of Na^+ and Ca^{2+} through
reverse mode of the Na^+/Ca^{2+} exchanger (NCX) (Kirischuk et al. 2012). The
reversal potential of NCX in astrocytes is set at levels close to the resting
membrane potential (Reyes et al. 2012); therefore NCX can quickly switch into
reverse mode in response to small $[Na^+]_i$ increases and/or depolarization
(Kirischuk et al. 2012; Paluzzi et al. 2007), as would be seen with VGSC
activation, causing an increase in $[Ca^{2+}]_i$.

Our work (**Chapter 2**) has shown that Nav1.5 plays an important role in an
in vitro model of glial injury via reverse action of NCX (Pappalardo et al. 2014b).
Astrocyte wound closure after mechanical injury is attenuated by
pharmacological treatment with TTX and KB-R7943 (at a dose that selectively
blocks reverse Na^+/Ca^{2+} exchange), and by knockdown of Nav1.5 mRNA. The
robust $[Ca^{2+}]_i$ response seen in astrocytes after mechanical injury, which

participates in the pathways leading to astrogliosis (Gao et al. 2013) is also attenuated by TTX, KB-R7943, and Nav1.5 knockdown (Pappalardo et al. 2014b). The upregulation of Nav1.5 in astrocytes *in situ* in animals with monophasic and CR EAE in correlation with increasing disease severity is consistent with these *in vitro* results. Together, these findings support the suggestion that Nav1.5 may be a potential target for modulation of astrogliosis after injury via effects on $[Ca^{2+}]_i$.

There is a growing body of evidence detailing the favorable effect of sodium channel blockade in animal models of neurological diseases, including EAE. Several sodium channel blockers have been studied, including phenytoin (Black et al. 2007; Lo et al. 2003), lamotrigine (Bechtold et al. 2006), carbamazepine (Black et al. 2007), safinamide and flecainide (Morsali et al. 2013). It is noteworthy that flecainide, a Class Ic cardiac anti-arrhythmic, has strong state-dependent effects on Nav1.5 (Ramos and O'Leary 2004). The present findings, along with others detailed here, raise the possibility that attenuation of reactive astrogliosis could contribute to the improved outcomes seen with sodium channel blockade. This study lends further insight to the suggestion that Nav1.5 can play a role in the response of astrocytes to neuroinflammatory pathologies, identifying this sodium channel as an attractive potential therapeutic target for modulating reactive astrogliosis *in vivo*.

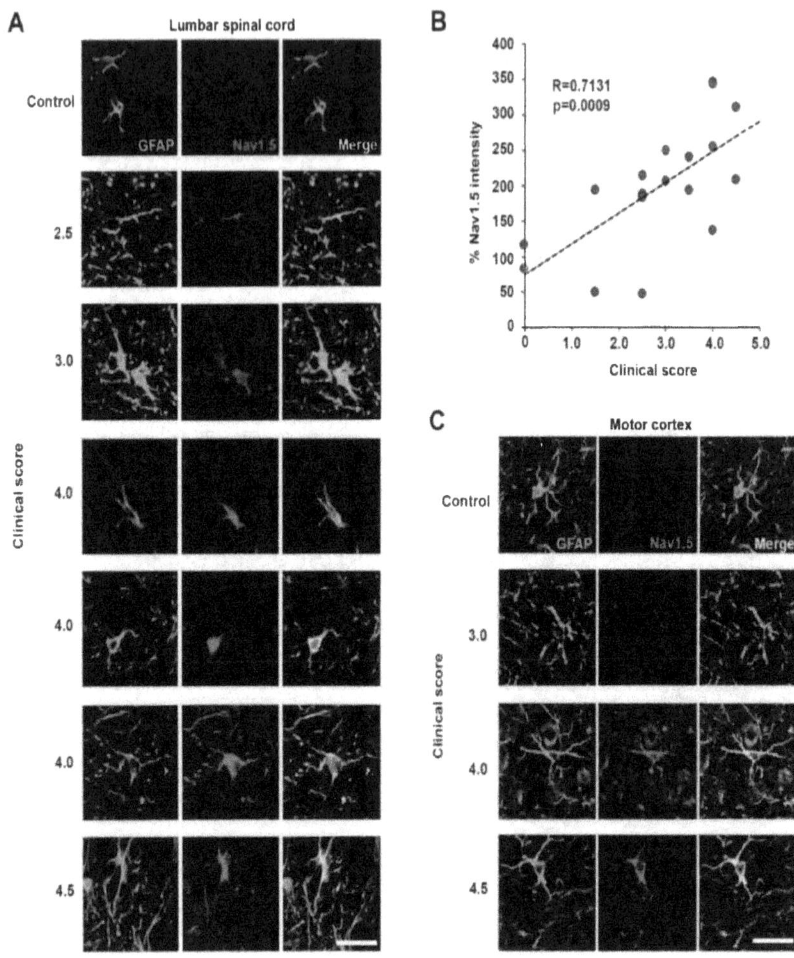

A
Lumbar spinal cord
Control
GFAP
Nav1.5
Merge
Clinical score
2.5
3.0
4.0
4.0
4.0
4.5
B
R=0.7131
p=0.0009
% Nav1.5 intensity
400
350
300
250
200
150
100
50
0
Clinical score
0   1.0   2.0   3.0   4.0   5.0
C
Motor cortex
Control
GFAP
Nav1.5
Merge
Clinical score
3.0
4.0
4.5

Figure 3.1 – Astrocytes in monophasic EAE upregulate Nav1.5 in the spinal cord and brain, in correlation with increasing disease severity. (A) GFAP-positive astrocytes (green) from the anterolateral white matter of the L1-L2 spinal cord of mice with monophasic EAE exhibit prominent Nav1.5 immunolabeling (red), which is upregulated in correlation with increasing clinical score (panels arranged top to bottom in order of increasing severity of disease). Control animal exhibits little astrocytic Nav1.5 immunolabeling (top panel). Merged images of GFAP and Nav1.5 are yellow. Scale bars, 25 µm. **(B)** Increasing clinical score is positively correlated with percent of astrocytic Nav1.5 upregulation as compared to control animals. Data represented as mean % intensity as compared to control animals **(C)** GFAP-positive astrocytes (green) from the motor cortex of mice with monophasic EAE exhibit prominent Nav1.5 immunolabeling (red), which is upregulated in correlation with increasing clinical score (panels arranged top to bottom in order of increasing severity of disease). Control animal exhibits little astrocytic Nav1.5 immunolabeling (top panel). Merged images of GFAP and Nav1.5 are yellow. Scale bar, 25 µm.

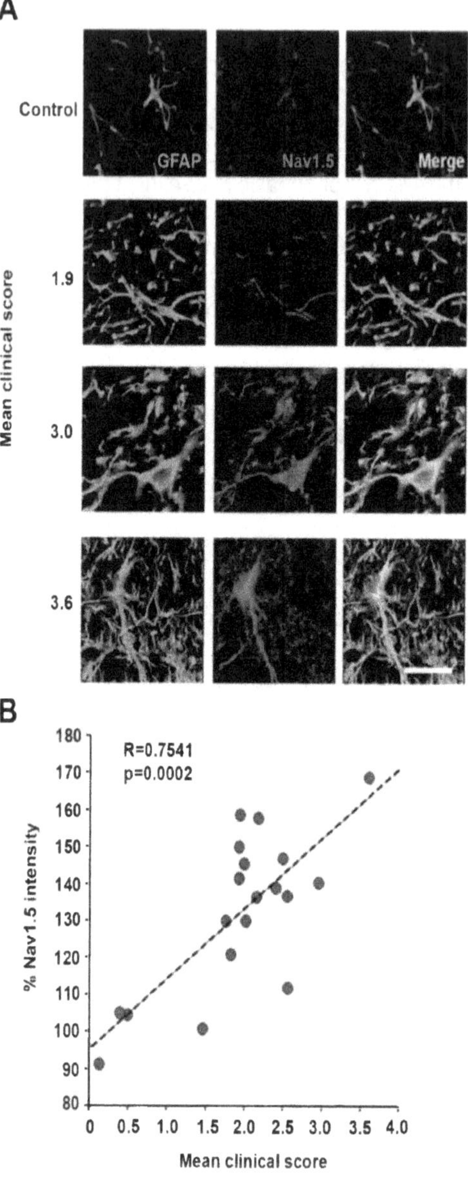

A
Control
GFAP
Nav1.5
Merge
Mean clinical score
1.9
3.0
3.6
B
180
170
160
150
140
130
120
110
100
90
80
% Nav1.5 intensity
R=0.7541
p=0.0002
0
0.5
1.0
1.5
2.0
2.5
3.0
3.5
4.0
Mean clinical score

Figure 3.2 – Astrocytes in chronic-relapsing EAE upregulate Nav1.5 in the anterolateral spinal cord, in correlation with increasing disease severity.
(A) GFAP-positive astrocytes (green) from the L1-L2 spinal cord of mice with chronic-relapsing EAE exhibit prominent Nav1.5 immunolabeling (red), which is upregulated in correlation with increasing mean clinical score (panels arranged top to bottom in order of increasing severity of disease). Control animal exhibits little astrocytic Nav1.5 immunolabeling (top panel). Merged images of GFAP and Nav1.5 are yellow. Scale bar, 25 µm. (B) Increasing mean clinical score is positively correlated with percent of astrocytic Nav1.5 upregulation as compared to control animals. Data represented as mean % intensity as compared to control animals.

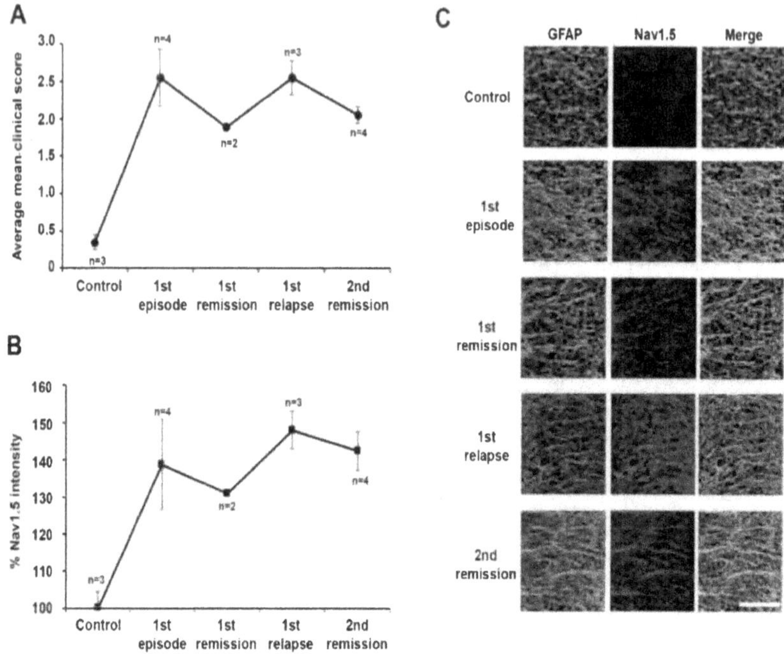

Figure 3.3 – Astrocytic Nav1.5 expression is attenuated during periods of remission in chronic-relapsing EAE. (A) MOG inoculation of Biozzi mice induced a chronic-relapsing form of EAE, with mean clinical scores of ~2.5 in the first episode and first relapse and ~1.8 and ~2.0 in the first and second remissions, respectively **(B)** Astrocytes within spinal cord white matter displayed Nav1.5 immunofluorescent signals that seemed to parallel the relapsing-remitting clinical course. **(C)** Quantification of Nav1.5 immunofluorescence in astrocytes in the chronic-relapsing phases is consistent with an upregulation of Nav1.5 in the first episode that is attenuated in the 1st remission, further upregulated in the 1st episode, and again attenuated in the 2nd remission. Data represented as mean % intensity as compared to control animals. Scale bar, 500 μm.

CHAPTER 4: NAV1.5 IN ASTROCYTES PLAYS A SEX-SPECIFIC ROLE IN CLINICAL OUTCOMES IN A MOUSE MODEL OF MULTIPLE SCLEROSIS

This chapter contains a modified version of material that appeared in the author's publication: Pappalardo LW, Samad OA, Liu S, Zwinger PJ, Black JA, Waxman SG (2018). Nav1.5 in astrocytes plays a sex-specific role in clinical outcomes in a mouse model of multiple sclerosis. GLIA: 1–14. https://doi.org/10.1002/glia.23470.

INTRODUCTION

Although circulating peripheral leukocytes are major effectors of CNS inflammation, there is increasing focus on CNS-intrinsic cells, which play essential roles in recruiting and regulating leukocytes at sites of CNS insults. Among CNS-intrinsic cells, astrocytes are now emerging as cells that can exert either potent pro-inflammatory functions or protective anti-inflammatory functions, as regulated by specific signaling inputs (Sofroniew 2015a).

Multiple sclerosis (MS) is an autoimmune disease of the CNS characterized by inflammation, demyelination, and axonal loss, involving both peripheral immune cell infiltrate and activated CNS-resident cell populations (McFarland and Martin 2007; Sospedra and Martin 2005). Experimental autoimmune encephalomyelitis (EAE) is a widely employed animal model for MS and has been used to study both peripheral immune responses and neurodegenerative aspects of neuroinflammation (Croxford et al. 2011; Gold et al. 2006; Mix et al. 2010; Ransohoff 2012; Slavin et al. 2010). Like MS, EAE is a

T cell-mediated autoimmune disease in which perivascular T cells and B cells, followed by macrophages, enter the CNS, leading to areas of demyelination and axonal loss, which correlates with motor deficits in standard EAE clinical scores (Herz et al. 2010; Wujek et al. 2002). Astrocytes play an important role in both MS and EAE by orchestrating the immune response of both peripheral and CNS-intrinsic cells (Brambilla et al. 2014). Understanding the specific cellular mechanisms which regulate the infiltration of inflammatory cells into the CNS during neuroinflammation is crucial to the development of treatment strategies aiming to block inflammation and improve functional outcomes in autoimmune disease.

There is sexual dimorphism in human autoimmune diseases such as MS; females are affected at rates of 2-3 times that of males (Voskuhl and Gold 2012). MS onset is rare during the latter half of pregnancy, but the risk of developing MS is elevated in the post-partum period (Confavreux et al. 1998). In addition, while women exhibit a higher incidence of MS and a more robust immune response, male patients tend to demonstrate a more progressive disease course and higher morbidity (Dunn et al. 2015). These phenomena suggest that sex hormones are important in MS disease pathogenesis and activity. Consistent with these clinical observations, it is well-established that estrogens are neuroprotective in numerous animal disease models of the CNS, including MS. EAE improves during pregnancy and estrogen treatment exerts well-documented neuroprotective effects in EAE. Interestingly, it has been shown that astrocytes are key players in modulating the neuroprotective effects of estrogen ligand treatment in EAE through estrogen receptor α (ERα) signaling and subsequent

modulation of the immune response, particularly levels of infiltrating monocytes

(Giraud et al. 2010; Spence et al. 2011; Spence et al. 2013).

Astrocytes respond to injury and disease through astrogliosis, which is a

hallmark of neuroinflammation in diseases such as MS (Sofroniew 2009;

Sofroniew 2015b). Reactive astrogliosis plays a fundamental role in determining

tissue repair and outcome, thus a thorough understanding of the governing

molecular mechanisms is required for development of therapeutic targets.

Though astrocytes have classically been considered to be electrically

unexcitable, these cells express voltage-gated sodium channels (VGSCs)

(Pappalardo et al. 2016; Sontheimer et al. 1992; Sontheimer et al. 1996),

particularly isoform Nav1.5 (Black et al. 1998; Pappalardo et al. 2014a;

Pappalardo et al. 2014b). Notably, Black et al. demonstrated the presence of

Nav1.5 in human scarring astrocytes within acute and chronic MS lesions, which

was supported by similar observations in rodents (Pappalardo et al. 2014a),

suggesting a commonality of upregulated astrocytic Nav1.5 in CNS inflammation.

Despite the well-characterized expression of VGSCs in both rodent and human

astrocytes, the functional role of these VGSCs has remained unknown. Recent

work has shown that Nav1.5 plays an important role in an *in vitro* model of glial

injury by triggering reverse mode operation of the Na^+-Ca^{2+} exchanger (NCX)

(Pappalardo et al. 2014b). These results suggest Nav1.5 as a potential target for

the modulation of astrogliosis. Given the dynamic expression of VGSCs in rodent

astrocytes (MacFarlane and Sontheimer 1998; Sontheimer et al. 1991; Thio and

Sontheimer 1993), the upregulation of Nav1.5 in scarring astrocytes in both MS (Black et al. 2010) and EAE (Pappalardo et al. 2014a), and the functional role of Nav1.5 in astrogliosis *in vitro* (Pappalardo et al. 2014b), we examined a possible role of Nav1.5 to astrocyte function in an *in vivo* model of MS.

Here, we investigate whether Nav1.5 expression in astrocytes plays a role in the pathogenesis of EAE. We have created a conditional knockout of Nav1.5 in astrocytes and determined whether the loss of Nav1.5 affects the clinical course of EAE, focal macrophage and T cell infiltration, and diffuse activation of astrocytes. We show that deletion of Nav1.5 from astrocytes leads to significantly worsened clinical outcomes in EAE, with increased inflammatory infiltrate in both early and late stages of disease, in a sex-specific manner.

MATERIALS AND METHODS

Animals

Conditional *Cre-loxP* based strategies have been successfully employed to produce tissue-specific knockout of Nav1.6 (Levin et al. 2006) and Nav1.7 (Nassar et al. 2004). Nav1.5 conditional gene deletion or knockout (KO) from astrocytes (astrocyte Nav1.5 KO) was generated by crossing transgenic mice that express Cre-recombinase constitutively under regulation of the mouse glial fibrillary acid protein (mGFAP) promoter from the B6.Cg-Tg(Gfap-cre)77.6Mvs/J line (JAX, Bar Harbor, ME; stock No. 024098), with mice carrying a SCN5A gene flanked by *loxP* sites (Nav1.5$^{F/F}$; described below). The loxP sites surround a critical portion of exon 2 in SCN5A, which renders all known Nav1.5 splice isoforms nonfunctional in GFAP-Cre expressing cells. Previous constitutive GFAP-Cre lines have been of limited use to target astrocytes in adult mice as postnatal GFAP-expressing progenitor cells are the principal source of constitutive neurogenesis in the adult mouse forebrain (Garcia et al. 2004). However, the mGFAP-Cre 77.6 line is reported to have no Cre recombinase activity in postnatal adult neural stem cells (or their progeny) from the hippocampus nor other brain regions (Gregorian et al. 2009); thus this line is particularly useful for selective targeting of astrocytes in the brain and spinal cord. These mice show robust recombination in astrocytes in the spinal cord (Su et al. 2014), cortex (Niu et al. 2013), and cerebellum (Tao et al. 2011), with most recombined cells expressing astrocyte markers (95-98%). We duplicated these findings by crossing the previously described Cre reporter Rosa-tdTomato mouse line (Luche et al. 2007) with mGFAP-Cre 77.6 animals and confirming through immunocytochemistry that all tdT-expressing cells also expressed GFAP (data not shown).

For generation of the Nav1.5$^{F/F}$ mouse colony, C57BL/6N-derived embryonic stem (ES) cells containing a targeted mutation of the voltage-gated sodium channel Nav1.5 (SCN5A) gene were obtained from The European Conditional Mouse Mutagenesis Program (EUCOMM). The mutant allele (*tm1a*), has from 5' to 3', a *FRT* site, a β-galactosidase gene, a *loxP* site, a neomycin resistance (neo) cassette, a second *FRT* site, and *loxP* sites flanking exon 2. Correctly targeted ES cells were injected into C57BL/6J blastocysts (JAX; stock No. 000058). Of the resulting chimeric mice, those determined to have germline transmission were bred to *Flp* deleter mice (JAX: stock No. 005703) to remove the selection cassette and the final Nav1.5$^{F/F}$ mice were backcrossed for several generations to wild-type (WT) C57/BL6 mice (Envigo, South Easton, MA). The final colony is therefore of a coisogenic genetic background consisting of C57BL/6N and C57BL/6J. Genotyping of the Nav1.5$^{F/F}$ colony was performed with the following primers:

5'-ACAGAATTGGGATTAGGGTTAGGG-3'

5'-AGCACACACGGTCTGGGCTTTGAGG-3'

5'-CAACGGTTCTTCTGTTAGTCC-3',

with the WT allele measuring 559 base pairs and the loxP allele 657 base pairs **(Fig. 4.1)**.

The final astrocyte Nav1.5 KO colony were bred in pairs of male GFAP-Cre/+; Nav1.5$^{F/F}$ and female +/+; Nav1.5$^{F/F}$ mice, resulting in 50% GFAP-Cre/+; Nav1.5 $^{F/F}$ mice (KO) and 50% +/+; Nav1.5$^{F/F}$ littermate wild-type mice (WT). No behavioral abnormalities were observed within the colony. Both KO and WT animals performed identically during baseline EAE clinical scoring (before MOG immunization). Animals were maintained under standard conditions in a 12 h dark/light cycle with access to food and water ad libitum. All procedures were carried out in accordance with the guidelines of the National Institutes of Health and the IACUC of VA Connecticut Healthcare System, West Haven, CT.

To confirm the selectivity of Nav1.5 deletion in astrocytes during EAE, we assessed Nav1.5 expression by immunohistochemistry using double staining for GFAP (green) and Nav1.5 (red), examining tissues from animals of both genotypes at similar clinical EAE stages (clinical score, 3.5). As seen in **Fig. 4.2A,** compared to WT littermate mice (+/+; Nav1.5$^{F/F}$, top panel), mice lacking Nav1.5 within astrocytes (Cre/+; Nav1.5$^{F/F}$, bottom panel) exhibit attenuated Nav1.5 expression (red) in GFAP+ astrocytes (green) located in the dorsal horn of the lumbar spinal cord. Similarly, WT mice (**Fig. 4.2B**, top panel) have significantly increased Nav1.5 expression (red) within astrocytes (green) in the anterior white matter of the lumbar spinal cord as compared to Nav1.5 knockout mice (bottom panel). Of note, some astrocytes from Nav1.5 KO mice appear to have a simpler morphology compared to those from WT mice. It is possible that astrocyte morphological changes are governed in part by Nav1.5 and this is a point of future investigation.

EAE induction

Male and female astrocyte Nav1.5 KO and littermate control (WT) mice 6–9 weeks of age were injected subcutaneously in the flank with 200 µl of an emulsion of 300 µg of rat myelin-oligodendrocyte glycoprotein (MOG) 35–55 peptide (W. M. Keck Biotechnology Resource Center, Yale University) in incomplete Freund's adjuvant (IFA; Sigma, St Louis, MO) supplemented with 500 µg of Mycobacterium tuberculosis H37Ra (Difco, Detroit, MI), as described previously (Black et al. 2006; Pappalardo et al. 2014a). The MOG injection, with mycobacterium supplemented IFA, was repeated in the contralateral flank 1 week later. The mice also received an injection of 250 ng pertussis toxin (PTx) (Sigma) in 200 µl phosphate-buffered saline (PBS) intraperitoneally (i.p.) immediately after the first immunization with MOG and then again 48 h later. In agreement with previous descriptions, the mice developed a monophasic clinical course. A total of 80 mice (18 Cre/+; Nav1.5$^{F/F}$ female, 20 Cre/+; Nav1.5$^{F/F}$ male, 21 +/+; Nav1.5$^{F/F}$ female, and 21 +/+; Nav1.5$^{F/F}$ male) were injected over 4 independent experiments.

Clinical assessment

Immunized mice were observed daily and scored on a 0 to 5 clinical scale with increasing clinical score reflecting clinical worsening as follows: 1—flaccid tail; 2—abnormal righting reflex and/or abnormal gait in the absence of weakness; 3—partial hindlimb paralysis; 4—complete hindlimb paralysis; 5—moribund (Matthaei et al. 1989). We applied the scale in 0.5 increments, with daily scoring beginning 10 days post-EAE induction. To calculate total burden of disease, clinical scores were summed daily through the animal's lifespan. Mean clinical score was determined by averaging clinical scores for all sick days of each animal.

Tissue collection

Mice were sacrificed at either 18 days (early EAE) or 28 days (chronic EAE) from date of induction of EAE. Mice were anesthetized with ketamine/xylazine (80/5 mg/kg i.p.) and perfused through the heart with phosphate-buffered saline (PBS) and then with 4% paraformaldehyde (PFA) in 0.14 M Sorensen's phosphate buffer. Spinal cords and brains were carefully excised, cryoprotected with 30% sucrose in PBS and frozen.

Immunocytochemistry

Twelve μm transverse sections of lumbar spinal were sectioned on a cryostat and incubated simultaneously with primary antibodies [mouse anti-glial fibrillary acidic protein (GFAP), 1:1000, Covance, Princeton, NJ; rabbit anti-Nav1.5, 1:100, Alomone, Jerusalem, Israel; rabbit anti-ionized calcium-binding adapter molecule 1 (Iba1), 1:1000, Wako, Richmond, VA; AlexaFluor® 647 rat anti-mouse CD3 molecular complex, 1:100, BD Biosciences, San Jose, CA] overnight at 4° C on a rotating shaker. Sections were rinsed 5 times with phosphate-buffered saline (PBS) and incubated with secondary antibodies [donkey anti-mouse immunoglobulin G-Alexa Fluor 488, 1:500, Invitrogen, Grand

Island, NY; donkey anti-rabbit immunoglobulin G Cy3, 1:500, Jackson, West

Grove, PA] overnight. Slides were rinsed with PBS and coverslips were mounted

with Aqua Poly mount (Polysciences, Warrington, PA). Control experiments were

performed with the omission of the primary antibodies and only background

labeling was observed.

Data acquisition and analysis

Multiple images of astrocyte Nav1.5 knockout and control tissues were

acquired with a Nikon C1*si* confocal microscope (Nikon USA, Melville, NY)

operating under identical gain settings with frame lambda (sequential) mode and

saturation indicator activated to prevent possible bleed-through between

channels. For quantitative analysis of GFAP, CD3, and Iba1 immunolabeling,

Image J software was utilized. Low magnification (20×) images of the lumbar

spinal cord were selected for analysis. Regions of interest for mean RGB

intensity analysis were created by manually outlining individual areas of lumbar

spinal cord, including total, white matter, gray matter, and dorsal regions. Multiple

images for each animal were taken, quantified, and averaged. Values were

normalized to RGB intensity of total spinal cord in 28 d WT animals. Twenty-

three female mice (5 WT and 5 KO at 18 d; 6 WT and 7 KO at 28 d) were

included in histological analysis. Images were composed and processed to

enhance contrast in the figures in Adobe Photoshop, with identical settings for

the different conditions.

Statistical methods

Data are presented as mean ± SEM from n determinations as indicated. Differences in EAE clinical scores were determined by repeated-measures one-way ANOVA. For comparison of total disease burden and mean clinical scores, data were analyzed with an unpaired Student t-test followed by Tukey's honest significance test. All statistics relating to clinical outcomes were performed with Origin 9.0 (Origin Lab Corporation, Northampton, MA). Significance was reached if p <0.05.

For differences in histological outcomes between EAE groups, data were analyzed with an unpaired Student t-test followed by Tukey's honest significance test in Origin 9.0. To assess histological correlation between GFAP, CD3, and Iba1 immunolabeling and animal clinical status, and Iba1 and GFAP immunolabeling, correlation coefficients (Spearman for normally distributed data; Pearson for nonparametric data) and two-tailed p-values were calculated with GraphPad Prism (GraphPad Software, La Jolla, CA). p<0.05 was considered to represent a significant difference.

RESULTS

Nav1.5 deletion from astrocytes during EAE leads to more severe clinical disease

To determine whether Nav1.5 in astrocytes plays a role in EAE, we compared standard EAE clinical scores in astrocyte Nav1.5 KO mice versus WT littermates. As seen in **Fig. 4.3A**, compared to WT mice (blue line), mice lacking Nav1.5 within astrocytes (red line) develop significantly more severe monophasic EAE over time, as indicated by clinical score (p=0.0110; n=80, 4 experiments,). Severity of disease was further measured by total disease burden (**Fig. 4.3B**; 35.9 ± 3.7 vs. 51.9 ± 3.4, p=0.0208) and mean clinical score (**Fig. 4.3C**; 1.9 ± 1.3 vs. 2.5 ± 0.1, p=0.0093), with Nav1.5 KO mice having significantly worse outcomes in both measurements compared to WT mice.

EAE clinical outcomes are sex-specific

Given the well-established sexual dimorphism in MS and the central role of astrocytes in estrogen-mediated neuroprotection in animal models of MS, we examined whether the observed clinical differences in EAE between astrocyte Nav1.5 KO and WT mice were sex-specific. Interestingly, male WT mice (**Fig. 4.4A**, purple line) and male astrocyte Nav1.5 KO mice (**Fig. 4.4A**, orange line) display no significant difference in daily EAE clinical scores (p=0.5678; n=41, 4 experiments), total disease burden (**Fig. 4.4B**; 48.4 ± 6.1 vs. 52.2 ± 3.4, p=0.5337), nor mean clinical scores (**Fig. 4.4C**; 2.6 ± 0.2 vs. 2.8 ± 0.1, p=0.4839) over course of disease. However, compared to female WT mice (**Fig. 4.4D**, yellow line), female mice lacking Nav1.5 in astrocytes (**Fig. 4.4D**, green line) develop significantly more severe monophasic EAE over time, as indicated by clinical score (p=0.0041; n=39, 3 experiments). Female WT mice (yellow) have significantly decreased overall disease burden (**Fig. 4.4E**; 30.5 ± 3.6 vs. 50.3 ± 5.4, p=0.0044) and decreased mean clinical score (**Fig. 4.4F**; 1.5 ± 0.2 vs. 2.4 ± 0.2 p=0.0020) over the EAE experiment compared to female astrocyte Nav1.5 KO mice (green). A summary of EAE clinical outcomes across all four groups is presented in **Fig. 4.5**.

Female Nav1.5 astrocyte knockout mice display increased CNS inflammatory markers in both early and chronic EAE

To understand how Nav1.5 in astrocytes alters the clinical course of EAE disease in female mice, we sacrificed mice during early disease (18 days) and chronic disease (28 days) to assess immune response. The effector phase of EAE disease involves the extravasation of activated myelin-specific T cells through the blood-brain barrier (BBB) and into perivascular spaces in the spinal cord. Here, the T cells encounter resident cells, resulting in further stimulation of pro-inflammatory cytokines and chemokines that mediate a secondary influx of other peripheral inflammatory cells including mononuclear phagocytes. We therefore assessed astrogliosis and immune infiltrates in the lumbar spinal cord of astrocyte Nav1.5 KO and WT female mice by immunofluorescence using GFAP (green) to mark astrogliosis, a T lymphocyte marker (CD3, blue), and a macrophage/microglia marker (Iba1, red) (**Fig. 4.6A**).

In general, there was increased astrogliosis, as indicated by GFAP immunolabeling, and immune cell infiltration, as indicated by CD3 and Iba1 immunolabeling, in KO mice compared to WT mice (**Fig. 4.6B-G**). Nav1.5 astrocyte KO mice (**Fig. 4.6B, C**, dark green) display an overall trend towards increased astrogliosis, as measured by GFAP expression, compared to WT mice (light green), particularly in the gray matter of the lumbar spinal cord 28 days post-EAE induction (102 ± 4 vs. 66 ± 11 % GFAP intensity, p=0.0170). Furthermore, knockout mice (**Fig. 4.6D**, dark blue) show increased CD3+ T cell infiltration in lumbar spinal cord white matter in early EAE (18 days) compared to WT mice (light blue) (175 ± 15 vs. 124 ± 17 % CD3 intensity), p=0.0456). There is no statistically significant difference in T cell infiltration at more chronic EAE time points (28 days) (**Fig. 4.6E**; p=0.2317). Finally, in chronic EAE, Nav1.5 astrocyte KO mice (**Fig. 4.6G**, dark red) have significantly increased numbers of Iba1+ macrophages/microglia in white and gray matter lumbar spinal cord compared to WT mice (light red) (213 ± 25 vs. 119 ±31 % Iba1 intensity, p=0.0468 and 134 ± 9 vs. 89 ± 16, Iba1 intensity, p=0.0387, respectively). There is no statistically significant difference in Iba1+ cell infiltration between WT and KO mice in early EAE (**Fig. 4.6F**; p=0.1944).

GFAP immunolabeling correlates with disease burden in female wild-type and astrocyte Nav1.5 knockout mice in early and chronic EAE

To further investigate the effects of Nav1.5 deletion on astrocyte functioning in EAE, we assessed the correlation of astrogliosis with disease severity, as inflammation is a key driver in EAE clinical scores (Brambilla et al., 2014). Astrogliosis, as indicated by GFAP immunolabeling, positively correlates with total disease burden of female mice in early (18 d) and chronic (28 d) EAE disease (**Fig. 4.7A**) in both control (**Fig. 4.7B**) and astrocyte Nav1.5 KO (**Fig. 4.7C**) animals across all regions of the lumbar spinal cord.

Iba1 immunolabeling in chronic EAE correlates with disease burden and GFAP immunolabeling in female wild-type but not astrocyte Nav1.5 knockout mice

To further explore the mechanism underlying differences in inflammation and clinical course between female WT and astrocyte Nav1.5 KO mice, we examined the correlation between levels of inflammation and clinical disease burden, focusing on areas where there was a statistically significant difference in inflammation between WT and KO mice (**Fig. 4.6C, D, G**). Interestingly, while levels of inflammation correlated with disease burden in WT animals, inflammatory infiltrate was either not significantly correlated, or inversely correlated with clinical disease burden in astrocyte Nav1.5 KO animals. In WT animals with chronic EAE, macrophage and microglial infiltration (Iba1) positively correlates with total disease burden in both white and gray matter of the lumbar spinal cord (**Fig. 4.8A, B, C**). In contrast, mice lacking Nav1.5 in astrocytes display an inverse correlation between macrophage/microglia activity and severity of disease in chronic EAE in both white and gray matter lumbar spinal cord (**Fig. 4.8D, E, F**).

Similarly, in WT mice with chronic EAE, macrophage and microglial activity (Iba1) positively correlates with astrogliosis (GFAP) in both white and gray matter of the lumbar spinal cord **(Fig. 4.9A, B, C).** In contrast, mice lacking Nav1.5 in astrocytes exhibit no significant correlation between macrophage/microglia infiltration and astroglial activity in chronic EAE in both white and gray matter lumbar spinal cord **(Fig. 4.9D, E, F)**. Collectively, these data point to a possible role of Nav1.5 in astrocytes in regulating the activity of activated macrophages/microglia in EAE.

We chose to display histological images and analysis only from female mice in this study, as the significant differences in EAE clinical outcomes were only observed between Nav1.5 KO and WT females. We did additionally process and examine tissue from the two male cohorts. There was no significant difference in GFAP, Iba1, or CD3 immunolabeling between male WT and male KO mice. The immunolabeling intensity in males is comparable to that of female Nav1.5 KO mice (data not shown).

In summary, these histopathological studies show that female Nav1.5 astrocyte KO mice display increased CNS inflammation in both early and chronic EAE and astrogliosis correlates with disease burden in female control and astrocyte Nav1.5 KO mice in early and chronic EAE. Additionally, monocyte reactivity in chronic EAE correlates with disease burden and astrogliosis in female control but not astrocyte Nav1.5 knockout mice, suggesting possible dysregulation of the immune response in mice lacking astrocytic Nav1.5.

4.4   DISCUSSION

By selectively removing sodium channel Nav1.5 from astrocytes, we found that Nav1.5 expression in astrocytes is functionally significant in EAE. Interestingly, this is a sex-specific phenomenon, with only female Nav1.5 astrocyte KO mice displaying significantly worsened clinical outcomes compared to female WT mice in EAE. Removal of Nav1.5 in astrocytes leads to increased inflammation in female mice with EAE, including increased astroglial response and infiltration of T cells and phagocytic monocytes, together consistent with more severe EAE clinical scores. Additionally, we found evidence suggesting possible dysregulation of the immune response – particularly with regard to infiltrating macrophages and activated microglia – in female Nav1.5 KO mice compared to controls.

Astrogliosis in response to CNS inflammation is context-dependent and plays an integral role in disease course, as astrocytes are intimately associated with and signal to blood vessels (Iadecola and Nedergaard 2007) and regulate leukocyte trafficking and inflammation in the CNS (Brosnan and Raine 2013; Rothhammer and Quintana 2015). Even in MS, which is classically considered a primarily T cell-dependent autoimmune neurodegenerative disease, astrocytes play a primary role in pathology. In acute active MS lesions, hypertrophic astrocytes are one of the earliest histopathological signs and perivascular astrocytes, which participate in formation of the blood-brain barrier (BBB), are highly affected in MS (Brosnan and Raine 2013). Astrocytes produce many pro-inflammatory chemokines and cytokines, as well as reactive oxygen species

(ROS) *in vitro*, consistent with a pro-inflammatory role, but also release anti-inflammatory cytokines and ROS scavengers, suggesting a role in attenuating inflammation (Dong and Benveniste 2001; Nair et al. 2008). It has been suggested that in EAE, astrocyte functioning may restrict neurotoxic inflammation. Astrocytes form borders (*glia limitans*) that separate neural from non-neural tissue along perivascular spaces, meninges and lesions in the CNS (Sofroniew 2015a). Numerous studies show that scar-forming reactive astrocytes form barriers essential in restricting leukocyte migration from areas of damaged tissue into neighboring healthy tissue (Bush et al. 1999; Faulkner et al. 2004; Herrmann et al. 2008; Li et al. 2008; Myer et al. 2006; Okada et al. 2006). In EAE, astrocyte loss-of-function studies show exacerbated disease course and inflammation (Liedtke et al. 1998; Toft-Hansen et al. 2011; Voskuhl et al. 2009).

Conversely, a more specific, pro-inflammatory role of astrocytes in orchestrating the immune response in EAE was recently reported: knockout of astrocytic transcription factor NF-κB resulted in reduced disease severity and improved functional recovery (Brambilla et al. 2009b), which the authors attributed to a reduction in peripheral immune cell infiltration into the CNS due to reduced immune cell mobilization from the periphery, diminished ability of T cells to produce pro-inflammatory cytokines, and reduced number of total and activated microglia (Brambilla et al. 2014; Brambilla et al. 2009b). Taken together, these findings indicate that while proper astrocyte functioning is crucial in regulating and limiting neuroinflammation, production of certain cytokines and chemokines may exert pro-inflammatory effects in specific contexts (Sofroniew 2014). Thus, astrocytes play complex roles in regulating CNS inflammation.

While there has been previous investigation into the roles of VGSCs in glia *in vitro* (Pappalardo et al. 2016; Sontheimer et al. 1992), this is the first study examining the functional role of glial VGSCs in a disease model *in vivo*. We have previously shown that Nav1.5 plays an important role in an *in vitro* model of glial injury by triggering reverse operation of the Na^+-Ca^{2+} exchanger (NCX), leading to fluctuations in $[Ca^{2+}]_i$, likely affecting downstream astrocyte functions such as process extension and proliferation, which contribute to wound closure **(Chapter 2)** (Pappalardo et al. 2014b). It is interesting that *in vitro*, blockade or knockdown of Nav1.5 attenuated the glial response to injury, while in EAE, lack of Nav1.5 in astrocytes resulted in increased astroglial response (i.e. increased GFAP expression), particularly in the lumbar spinal cord gray matter of KO animals in chronic EAE. It is important to note that the two studies invoke different methods of producing astrogliosis – one using an *in vitro* model of traumatic injury and the other a model of *in vivo* CNS autoimmune/inflammatory disease – which might account for the differential effects of Nav1.5 on astrocyte function. It is additionally important to consider potential developmental effect, as the Cre line used in this study was constitutive. It is possible that Nav1.5 plays a crucial role in astrocyte development and that decreased levels of Nav1.5 lead to dysfunctional astrocytes that are unable to properly maintain a normal response to neuroinflammation. Alternatively, it is possible that loss of Nav1.5 in astrocytes during development adversely affects the migration of neurons or other cells within the CNS. Nonetheless, irrespective of the underlying mechanisms, it is clear that Nav1.5 plays a role in shaping the response of astrocytes to injury and disease both *in vitro* and *in vivo* and may represent a potential therapeutic target for the modulation of astrogliosis.

We observed marked sexual dimorphism in this study: overall, while mice lacking Nav1.5 in astrocytes fared significantly worse than WT animals, the effect was predominately female. A likely mechanism underlying this observation may involve differences in sex hormones, namely estrogens. There are significant gender differences in the prevalence of human autoimmune diseases, including systemic lupus erythematosus (SLE), rheumatoid arthritis (RA), Graves' disease, and MS, all of which are more prevalent in females (Spence and Voskuhl 2012). During the third trimester of pregnancy, circulating levels of estrogens are at their peak, which correlates with a reduction in relapse rates among women with MS. Post-partum, levels of estrogens drop markedly and correlate with a significant increase in relapse rates during the 3-6 months after delivery (Confavreux et al. 1998). In addition, some studies demonstrate that pregnancy may offer long term protection to women with MS via regulation of the immune response (Runmarker and Andersen 1995; Verdru et al. 1994). Finally, while women exhibit a higher incidence of MS and a more robust immune response, male patients tend to demonstrate a more progressive disease course and higher morbidity (Dunn et al. 2015). These sex differences are also found in EAE animal models, depending on strain (Papenfuss et al. 2004). Together, these observations indicate that sex hormones are important in MS disease pathogenesis and activity.

Consistent with the clinical observations, it is now well-established that estrogens are neuroprotective in numerous animal disease models of the CNS, including MS. EAE in guinea pigs, rats, rabbits, and mice improves during pregnancy and estrogen treatment exerts neuroprotective effects in EAE in both sexes of mice and multiple strains via numerous anti-inflammatory effects in the peripheral immune system (Laffont et al. 2015; Voskuhl and Gold 2012). Since estrogens are lipophilic and thus able to cross the BBB, CNS cell populations are potential estrogen targets (Wise et al. 2001). Two main estrogen receptor (ER) subtypes – the nuclear receptors ERα and ERβ – are known to exist (Arevalo et al. 2015). The neuroprotective effect of estrogen treatment in EAE has been shown to depend on the presence of ERα but not ERβ (Liu et al. 2003; Polanczyk et al. 2003), and stimulation of ERα is sufficient to confer protection in EAE (Elloso et al. 2005; Morales et al. 2006). Additionally, it has been shown that expression of ERα in the peripheral immune system is dispensable for the estrogenic neuroprotective effect (Garidou et al. 2004), drawing attention to potential CNS targets of estrogens.

Astrocytes are known to express ERs (Garcia-Ovejero et al. 2002) and removal of reactive astrocytes has been reported to worsen EAE (Voskuhl et al. 2009). Indeed, it has recently been shown that astrocytes (but not neurons) are a key player in modulating the neuroprotective effects of estrogen ligand treatment in EAE through ERα signaling and subsequent immune response modulation

(Giraud et al. 2010; Spence et al. 2011; Spence et al. 2013). Specifically, induction of EAE in a conditional knockout of ERα from astrocytes renders ERα ligand treatment no longer protective from either T cell and macrophage CNS infiltration nor axonal loss (Spence et al., 2011). These observations are mediated at least in part by the effects of ERα signaling on astrocyte production of pro-inflammatory cytokines such as CCL2, which plays an important role in the recruitment of macrophages and T cells to the CNS during autoimmune disease (Spence et al., 2013; Kim et al., 2014). Thus, ERα expression on astrocytes is indispensable in providing estrogen ligand-mediated neuroprotection in EAE.

The present results are consistent with a possible role of Nav1.5 in modulating the neuroprotective effects of estrogen signaling in astrocytes. Mice lacking Nav1.5 in astrocytes show a significant increase in CNS inflammatory infiltrate consisting of both T cells and macrophages/microglia. This effect is primarily seen in female mice, suggesting a possible interaction of sex hormones and the functional role of Nav1.5 in astrocytes. Finally, while monocyte infiltration positively correlates with both astrogliosis and disease severity in control mice with chronic EAE, there is a loss of this correlation in astrocyte Nav1.5 KO mice, pointing to possible dysregulation of the immune response in EAE. While the mechanisms underlying a possible interaction between Nav1.5 and the neuroprotective effects of estrogen signaling in astrocytes require further investigation, it is interesting to note that studies have shown that estradiol regulates different functional parameters in astrocytes, such as intracellular Ca^{2+} levels (Chaban et al. 2004; Micevych et al. 2010). Similarly, Nav1.5 regulates

$[Ca^{2+}]_i$ levels in astrocytes *in vitro* (Pappalardo et al., 2014a), pointing to a potential point of mechanistic convergence.

Finally, there are many studies describing the favorable effect of sodium channel blockade in animal models of neuroinflammatory diseases: previous studies in EAE have shown reduction of axon loss and improved clinical status following treatment with a variety of voltage-gated sodium channel blockers including phenytoin (Black et al. 2007; Craner et al. 2005; Lo et al. 2002; Lo et al. 2003), lamotrigine (Bechtold et al. 2006), carbamazepine (Black et al. 2007), safinamide (Morsali et al. 2013), and flecainide (Bechtold et al. 2004; Bechtold et al. 2005; Morsali et al. 2013). Aside from astrocytes, peripheral and CNS-intrinsic immune cells involved in EAE also express sodium channels, including microglia (Black et al. 2009; Black and Waxman 2012; Craner et al. 2005; Korotzer and Cotman 1992; Nicholson and Randall 2009; Persson et al. 2014; Schmidtmayer et al. 1994), macrophages (Black et al. 2013; Carrithers et al. 2011; Carrithers et al. 2009; Carrithers et al. 2007; Craner et al. 2005; Schmidtmayer et al. 1994), and lymphocytes (DeCoursey et al. 1985; Decoursey et al. 1987; Fraser et al. 2008; Lai et al. 2000; Lo et al. 2012). Thus, it has been proposed that the clinical protection afforded by sodium channel-blocking agents is in part attributable to the modulation of the response of immune cells and/or glial cells to neuroinflammation via sodium channel blockade (Morsali et al. 2013).

Given this large body of evidence documenting a favorable effect of sodium channel blockade in preclinical MS models, it is critical to account for the surprising discrepancy between these previous findings and our observation that lack of sodium channel Nav1.5 in astrocytes leads to increased T cell and

macrophage/microglia infiltration and significantly worsened clinical outcomes in

EAE. This worsened effect was only observed in female mice – male mice

lacking Nav1.5 in astrocytes did not exhibit significantly worse outcomes than

male WT mice. Importantly, it appears that all previous studies demonstrating a

favorable effect of sodium channel blockade in EAE were performed using male

rodents (Bechtold et al. 2004; Bechtold et al. 2006; Black et al. 2007; Craner et

al. 2005; Lo et al. 2002; Lo et al. 2003; Morsali et al. 2013). It is possible that

EAE studies including both male and female animals would yield less favorable

effects of nonselective sodium channel blockers. Consistent with this, a recent

study examining the effects of selective sodium channel blockade (Nav1.2,

Nav1.4, Nav1.6) in female mice found significantly worsened clinical outcomes in

EAE (Stevens et al. 2013). Interestingly, the two clinical trials to-date

investigating the neuroprotective potential of sodium channel blockers in

neuroinflammation (lamotrigine in secondary progressive MS, phenytoin in acute

optic neuritis) included a majority of female patients (73% female both studies)

and yielded less positive results than perhaps expected (Kapoor et al. 2010;

Raftopoulos et al. 2016). Whether this is attributable to sodium channel

functioning in astrocytes is not clear. It seems likely that sodium channels play

cell-specific roles, conferring both beneficial and detrimental effects to outcomes

in neurological disease. It is also possible, though speculative at this time, that

sodium channel blockade has differing therapeutic benefit in a sex-dependent

manner. Additional *in vivo* studies are of importance for determination of the therapeutic implications of targeting glial sodium channels in neurological

disorders.

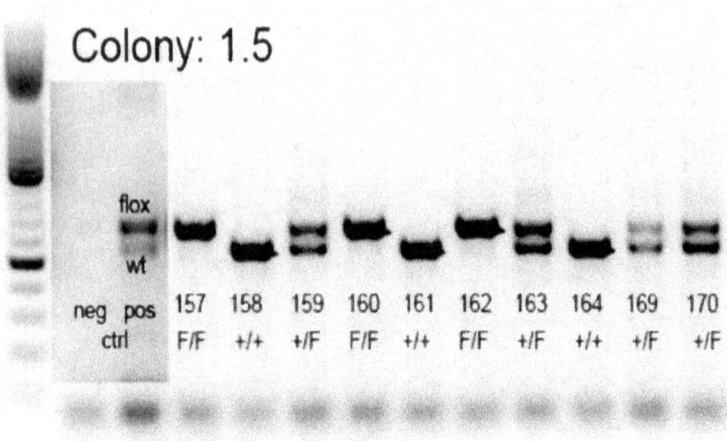

Figure 4.1 – Characterization of Nav1.5$^{F/F}$ mouse. PCR demonstrating three possible outcomes for Nav1.5$^{F/F}$ offspring. Wild-type SCN5A allele is 559 base pairs, whereas mutant SCN5A containing loxP sites is 490 base pairs.

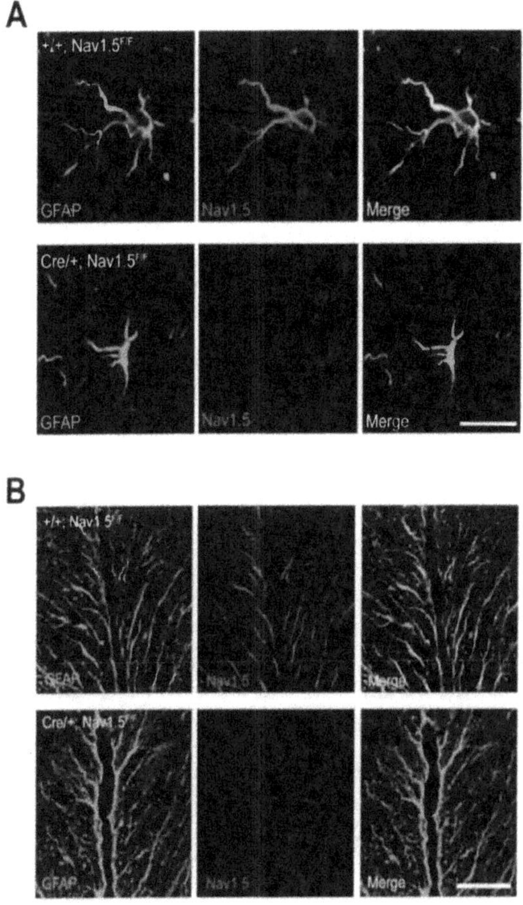

Figure 4.2 – Nav1.5 astrocyte knockout mice exhibit decreased Nav1.5 expression. (A) Compared to wild-type littermate mice (+/+; Nav1.5$^{F/F}$, top panel), mice lacking Nav1.5 in astrocytes (Cre/+; Nav1.5$^{F/F}$, bottom panel) exhibit attenuated Nav1.5 expression (red) in GFAP+ astrocytes (green) located in the dorsal horn of the lumbar spinal cord as evidenced by immunostaining. Scale bar, 50 µm. **(B)** WT mice (top panel) have significantly increased Nav1.5 expression (red) within astrocytes (green) in the anterior white matter of the lumbar spinal cord as compared to Nav1.5 KO mice (bottom panel). Images obtained from WT and KO female mice with equal clinical scores 28 days-post EAE immunization. Scale bar, 200 µm.

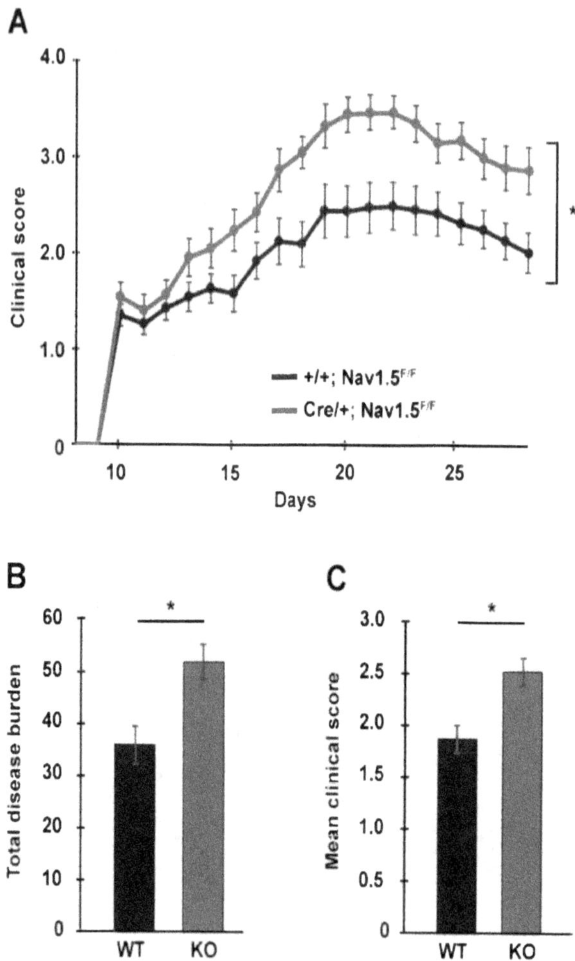

Figure 4.3 – Mice lacking astrocytic Nav1.5 develop more severe EAE. **(A)** Compared to wild-type littermate mice (+/+; Nav1.5$^{F/F}$; blue line), mice lacking Nav1.5 in astrocytes (Cre/+: Nav1.5$^{F/F}$; red line) develop significantly more severe monophasic EAE over time, as indicated by clinical score **(B)** Wild-type mice (WT; blue) have significantly decreased overall disease burden over a 28d EAE experiment compared to Nav1.5 astrocyte knockout mice (KO; red). **(C)** Wild-type mice (WT; blue) have significantly decreased mean clinical score over a 28 d EAE experiment compared to Nav1.5 astrocyte knockout mice (KO; red). Data represent n=80 mice over 4 separate experiments. *p<0.05.

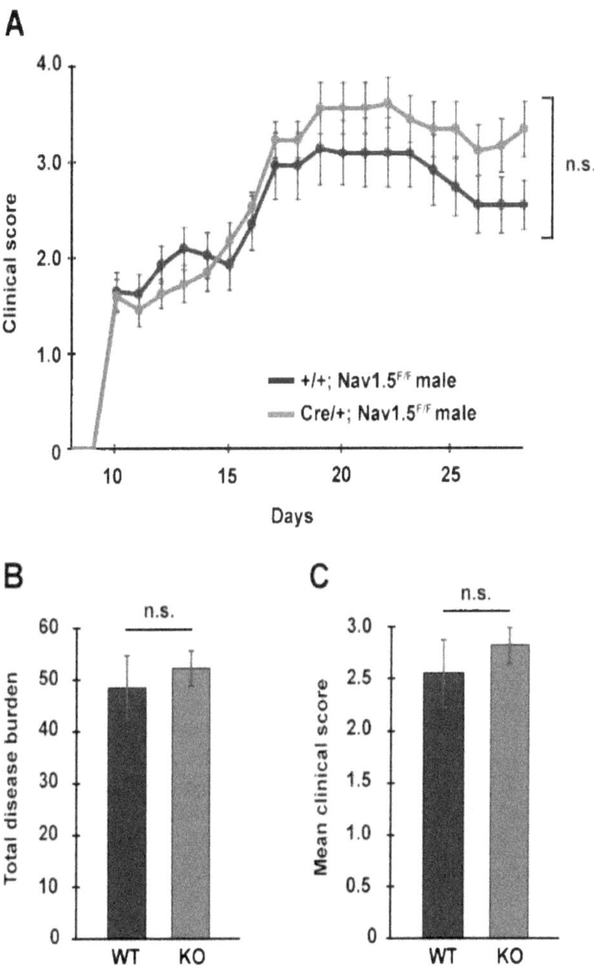

Figure 4.4 – EAE clinical outcomes in astrocyte Nav1.5 knockout mice are sex-specific. Male wild-type mice (+/+; Nav1.5$^{F/F}$; purple) and astrocyte Nav1.5 knockout mice (Cre/+: Nav1.5$^{F/F}$; orange) display no significant difference in **(A)** daily EAE clinical scores, **(B)** total disease burden, **(C)** nor mean clinical scores over course of disease. Data represent n=44 male mice over 4 separate experiments. n.s., not significant.

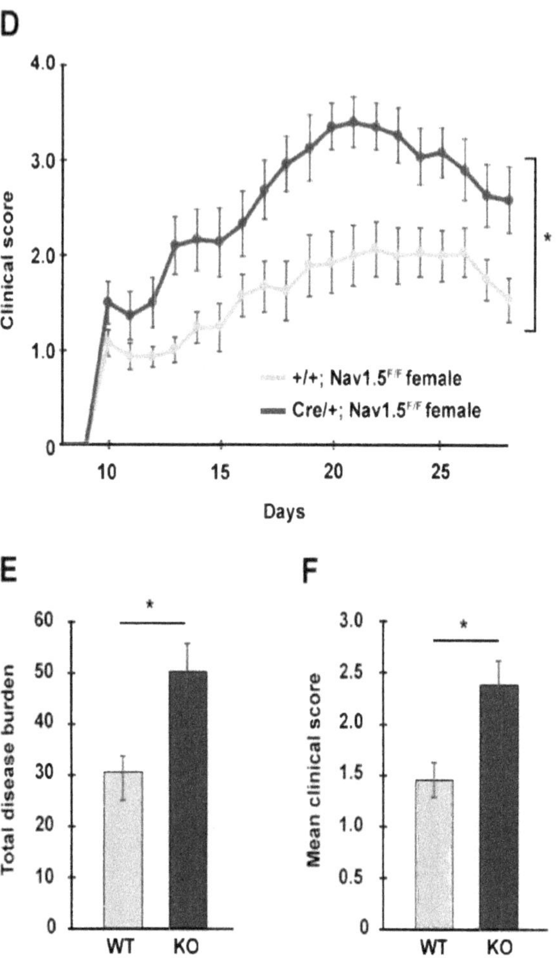

(D) Compared to female wild-type mice (+/+; Nav1.5$^{F/F}$; yellow line), female mice lacking Nav1.5 in astrocytes (Cre/+: Nav1.5$^{F/F}$; green line) develop significantly more severe monophasic EAE over time, as indicated by clinical score. Female wild-type mice (WT; yellow) have significantly decreased overall disease burden (E) and decreased mean clinical score (F) over a 28 d EAE experiment compared to female Nav1.5 astrocyte knockout mice (KO; green). Data represent n=39 female mice over 3 separate experiments. *p<0.05

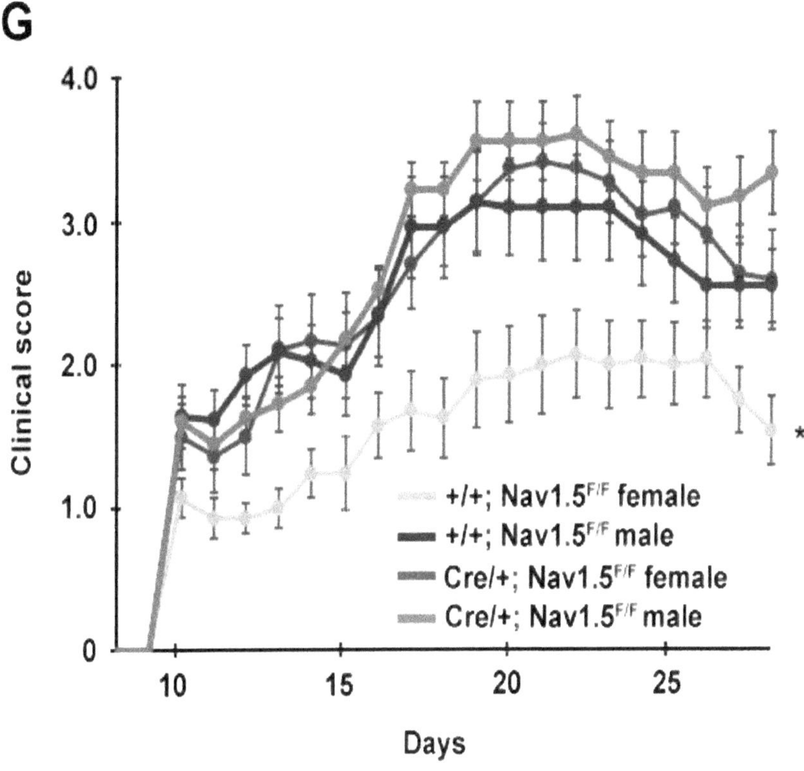

Figure 4.5 – Summary of EAE clinical outcomes in astrocyte Nav1.5 knockout mice. Male control mice (+/+; Nav1.5$^{F/F}$; purple line) and male astrocyte Nav1.5 knockout mice (Cre/+: Nav1.5$^{F/F}$; orange line) display no significant difference in daily EAE clinical scores. Female mice lacking Nav1.5 in astrocytes (Cre/+: Nav1.5$^{F/F}$; green line) develop significantly more severe monophasic EAE over time, as indicated by clinical score, equaling the disease severity of male mice from both groups, when compared to female wild-type mice (+/+; Nav1.5$^{F/F}$; yellow line), Data represent n=80 male and female mice over 4 separate experiments. *$p < 0.05$

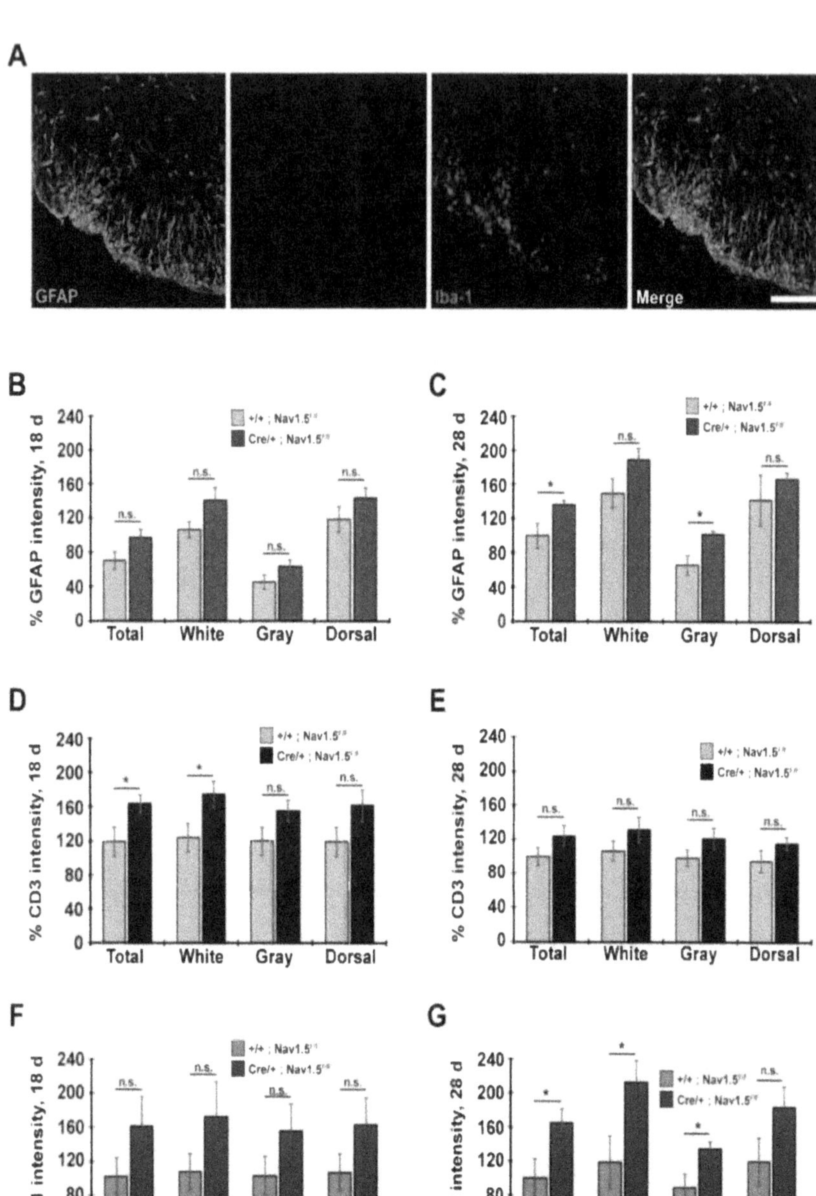

A
GFAP
Iba-1
Merge

B
% GFAP intensity, 18 d
+/+ ; Nav1.5
Cre/+ ; Nav1.5
n.s.
n.s.
n.s.
n.s.
240
200
160
120
80
40
0
Total
White
Gray
Dorsal

C
% GFAP intensity, 28 d
+/+ ; Nav1.5
Cre/+ ; Nav1.5
n.s.
n.s.
240
200
160
120
80
40
0
Total
White
Gray
Dorsal

D
% CD3 intensity, 18 d
+/+ ; Nav1.5
Cre/+ ; Nav1.5
n.s.
n.s.
240
200
160
120
80
40
0
Total
White
Gray
Dorsal

E
% CD3 intensity, 28 d
+/+ ; Nav1.5
Cre/+ ; Nav1.5
n.s.
n.s.
n.s.
n.s.
240
200
160
120
80
40
0
Total
White
Gray
Dorsal

F
% Iba-1 intensity, 18 d
+/+ ; Nav1.5
Cre/+ ; Nav1.5
n.s.
n.s.
n.s.
n.s.
240
200
160
120
80
40
0
Total
White
Gray
Dorsal

G
% Iba-1 intensity, 28 d
+/+ ; Nav1.5
Cre/+ ; Nav1.5
n.s.
240
200
160
120
80
40
0
Total
White
Gray
Dorsal

143

Figure 4.6 – Female Nav1.5 astrocyte knockout mice display increased CNS inflammation in both early and chronic EAE. **(A)** Example EAE lesion in anterior white matter of lumbar spinal cord showing robust astrogliosis (GFAP, green), T cell infiltration (CD3, blue) and Iba1-positive monocytes (red). Image obtained 18 days post-EAE immunization from Cre/+; Nav1.5$^{F/F}$ female mouse with a clinical score of 3.5. Scale bar, 200 µm. **(B), (C)** Nav1.5 astrocyte KO mice (dark green) have an overall trend towards increased astrogliosis, as measured by GFAP expression, compared to WT mice (light green), particularly in the gray matter of the lumbar spinal cord 28 days post-EAE induction. **(D), (E)** Cre/+; Nav1.5$^{F/F}$ mice (dark blue) show increased CD3+ T cell infiltration in lumbar spinal cord white matter in early EAE (18 days) compared to WT mice (light blue). There is no statistically significant difference in T cell infiltration at more chronic EAE time points (28 days). **(F), (G)** In chronic EAE (28 days), Nav1.5 astrocyte KO mice (dark red) have significantly increased numbers of Iba1+ macrophages/microglia in white and gray matter lumbar spinal cord compared to WT mice (light red). There is no statistically significant difference in Iba1+ cell infiltration between WT and KO mice in early EAE (18 days). Data represent n=23 female mice (6 WT and 7 KO at 18 d; 5 WT and 5 KO at 28 d). $*p<0.05$

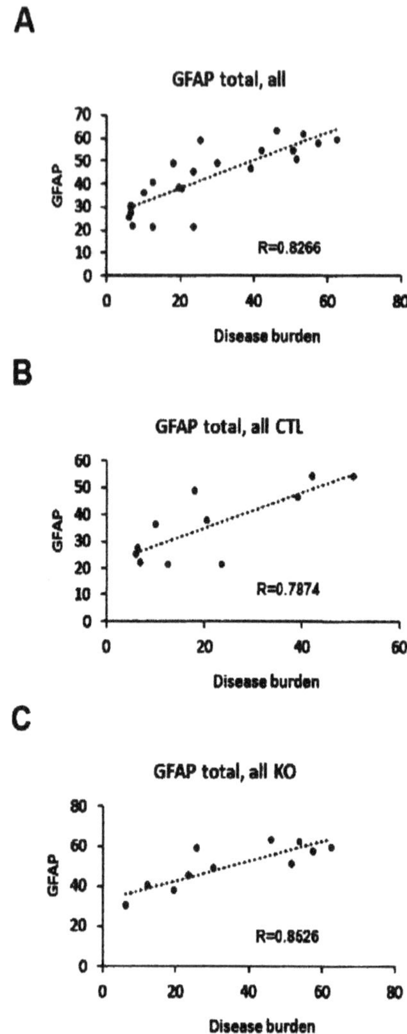

Figure 4.7 – Astrogliosis correlates with disease burden in female wild-type and astrocyte Nav1.5 knockout mice in early and chronic EAE. (A) Astrogliosis, as indicated by GFAP immunolabeling, positively correlates with total disease burden of female mice in early (18 d) and chronic (28 d) EAE disease in both control (**B**) and astrocyte Nav1.5 knockout (**C**) animals across all regions of the lumbar spinal cord. Data represent n=23 female mice (6 WT and 7 KO at 18 d; 5 WT and 5 KO at 28 d).

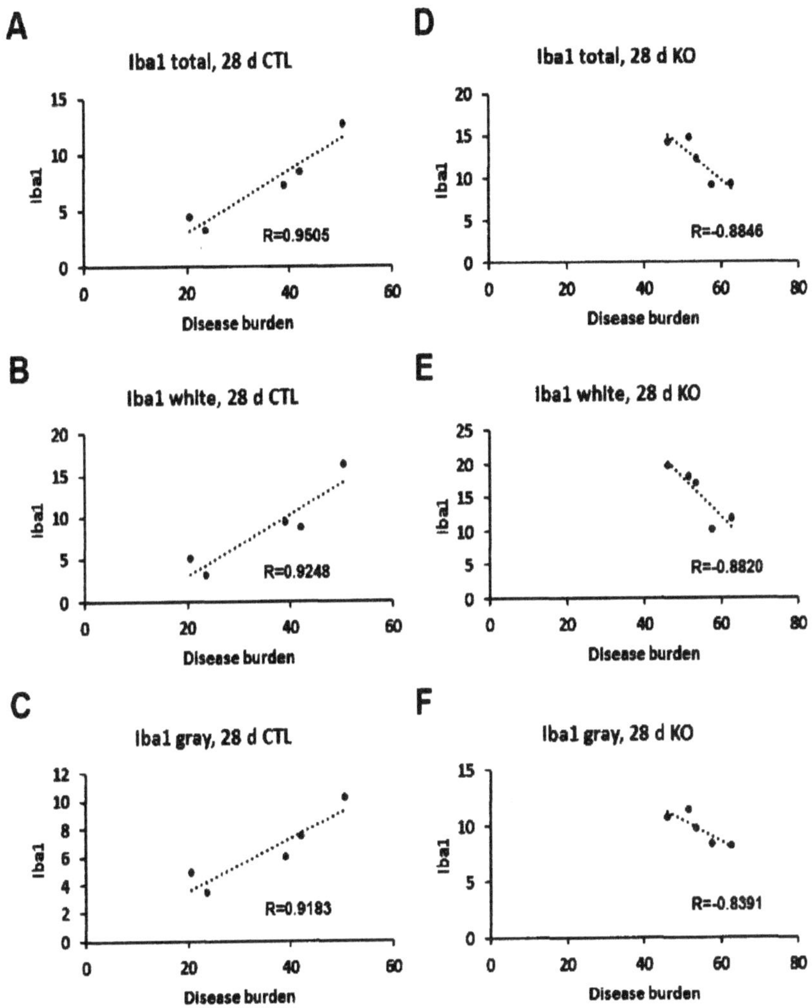

Figure 4.8 – Macrophage/microglia reactivity in wild-type EAE correlates with disease burden in control but not astrocyte Nav1.5 knockout mice. (A, B, C) In control mice with chronic EAE (28 d), macrophage and microglial infiltration (Iba1) positively correlates with total disease burden in both white and gray matter of the lumbar spinal cord. **(D, E, F)** In contrast, mice lacking Nav1.5 within astrocytes display an inverse correlation between macrophage/microglia activity and severity of disease in chronic EAE in both white and gray matter lumbar spinal cord. Data represent n=10 female mice (5 WT and 5 KO at 28 d).

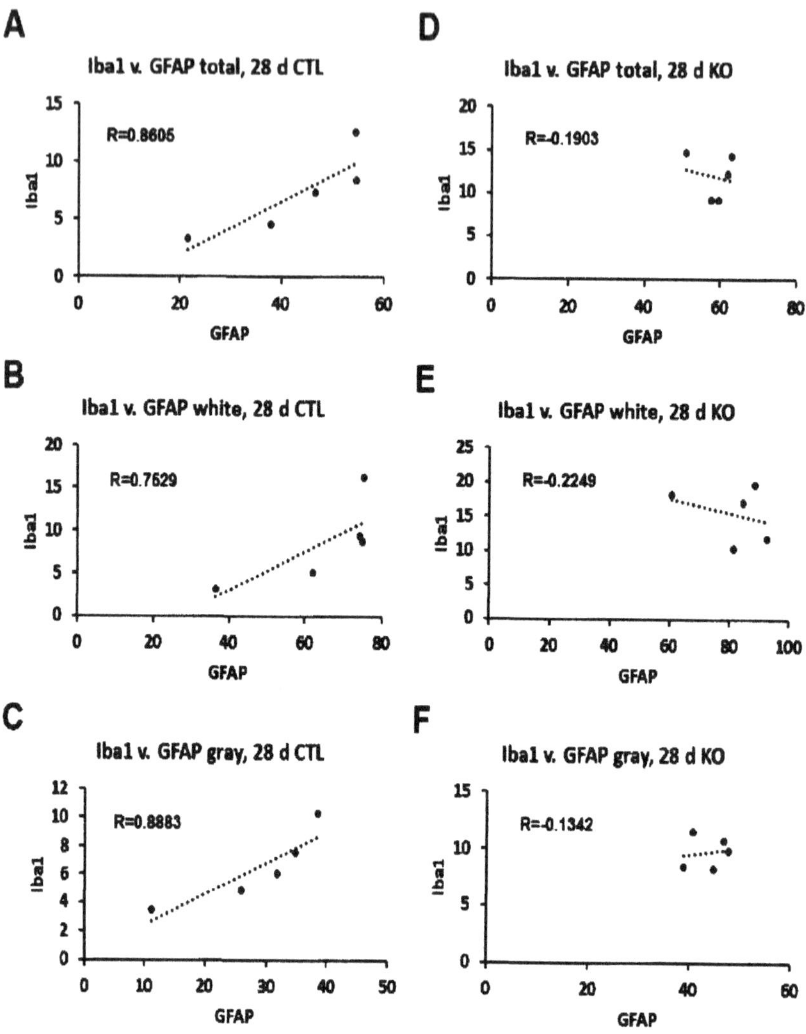

Figure 4.9 – Macrophage/microglia reactivity in chronic EAE correlates with astrogliosis in wild-type but not astrocyte Nav1.5 knockout mice. (A, B, C) Macrophage and microglial activity (Iba1) positively correlates with astrogliosis (GFAP) in control mice in both white and gray matter of the lumbar spinal cord in chronic EAE (28 d). **(D, E, F)** In contrast, mice lacking Nav1.5 within astrocytes exhibit no significant correlation between macrophage/microglia infiltration and astroglial activity in chronic EAE in both white and gray matter lumbar spinal cord. Data represent n=10 female mice (5 WT and 5 KO at 28 d).

5.1 SUMMARY

This works adds to the growing body of knowledge regarding the noncanonical function of voltage-gated sodium channels. We present here evidence supporting a contribution of sodium channel Nav1.5 to astrogliosis in an *in vitro* model of glial mechanical injury (**Chapter 2**). We further implicate fluctuations in $[Ca^{2+}]_i$ due to reverse operation of NCX, triggered by VGSC activity, as a mechanism by which Nav1.5 contributes to the response of astrocytes to mechanical injury. Our results establish a link between the activity of VGSCs and astrogliosis by way of alterations in $[Ca^{2+}]_i$. The detailed molecular mechanisms that control astroglial scarring following CNS insult are complex and an area of active investigation. Homeostatic functions of astrocytes by way of Na^+ and Ca^{2+} signaling play important roles in both physiological and pathological states (Parpura and Verkhratsky 2012). Here we show, in an *in vitro* model of mechanical injury to astrocytes, that voltage-gated sodium channel (VGSC) Nav1.5, traditionally viewed as a cardiac sodium channel, contributes to the astrocytic response to the insult via triggering reverse mode of the Na^+/Ca^{2+} exchanger (NCX). This study provides support for a contribution of VGSCs in the pathway leading to astrogliosis following mechanical injury.

Building upon previous work demonstrating the dynamic expression of VGSCs in rodent astrocytes (MacFarlane and Sontheimer 1998; Sontheimer et al. 1991; Thio and Sontheimer 1993), the upregulation of Nav1.5 in human scarring astrocytes (Black et al. 2010), and the functional role of Nav1.5 in glial scar formation *in vitro* (Pappalardo et al. 2014b), we also examined the temporal dynamics of Nav1.5 expression in scarring astrocytes in neuroinflammatory pathologies, with respect to disease severity and periods of relapse/remission (**Chapter 3**). We investigated the expression of astrocytic Nav1.5 in two mouse models of MS, monophasic experimental autoimmune encephalomyelitis (EAE) and chronic-relapsing EAE (CR EAE). We show that Nav1.5 upregulation correlates to disease severity and that Nav1.5 expression in astrocytes is modulated in parallel with periods of disease and remission.

Finally, to extend this work *in vivo*, we investigated whether Nav1.5 expression in astrocytes plays a role in the pathogenesis of EAE (**Chapter 4**). We created a conditional knockout of Nav1.5 in astrocytes and determined whether this affects the clinical course of EAE, focal macrophage and T cell infiltration, and diffuse activation of astrocytes. We show that deletion of Nav1.5 from astrocytes leads to significantly worsened clinical outcomes in EAE, with increased inflammatory infiltrate in both early and late stages of disease, in a sex-specific manner. Removal of Nav1.5 in astrocytes leads to increased inflammation in female mice with EAE, including increased astroglial response and infiltration of T cells and phagocytic monocytes. These cellular changes are consistent with more severe EAE clinical scores. Additionally, we found evidence suggesting possible dysregulation of the immune response – particularly regarding infiltrating macrophages and activated microglia – in female Nav1.5 KO mice compared to WT littermate controls.

These studies demonstrate the presence and upregulation of Nav1.5 in astrocytes of a murine model of MS and begin to elucidate the functional role of Nav1.5 in astrocytes *in vitro and in vivo*. This work is significant in that the results could expand current knowledge regarding the molecular mechanisms regulating effector functions of astrocytes *in vivo* and lend insight into future targets for the therapeutic modification of astrogliosis in disorders such as MS.

5.2 MOLECULAR MECHANISMS OF GLIAL SODIUM CHANNEL FUNCTION

While there is considerable evidence that sodium channels contribute to the regulation of physiological functions of glia, especially regarding the orchestrated response to CNS insult, there are currently limited data detailing the underlying mechanisms, which is an area of active investigation. It is likely that there are multiple molecular pathways; thus it is useful to consider the signaling cascades that have been suggested to link the activity of sodium channels to effector functions in other nonexcitable cells (Black and Waxman 2013), such as immune cells (Lo et al. 2012) and cancer cells (House et al. 2015). For example, blockade or knockdown of Nav1.5 inhibits the sustained Ca^{2+} influx required for the positive selection of CD4+/CD8+ T lymphocytes (Lo et al. 2012) and invasiveness of melanoma cells seems to rely on activation of Nav1.6, which increases intracellular Ca^{2+} release and invadopodia formation in those cells (Carrithers et al. 2009).

Although glia do not generate action potentials under physiological conditions, these cells can exhibit excitability by way of ionic fluxes, particularly in the form of $[Ca^{2+}]_i$ oscillations (Verkhratsky and Kettenmann 1996). Ca^{2+} dynamics participate in the regulation of microglial activation and multiple effector functions, including cell migration (Ifuku et al. 2007; Noda et al. 2013) and release of chemokines/cytokines and nitric oxide (Farber and Kettenmann 2006; Hoffmann et al. 2003; Ikeda et al. 2013). Astroglial $[Ca^{2+}]_i$ fluxes also modulate neuronal synapses, a phenomenon termed "gliotransmission" (Agulhon et al.

2008), and intracellular Ca^{2+} levels are critical for numerous cellular functions in astrocytes, including migration and proliferation (Parnis et al. 2013; Stanimirovic et al. 1995; Wang et al. 2010), both of which are processes involved in astrogliosis (Faulkner et al. 2004; Pappalardo et al. 2014b; Wanner et al. 2013). For example, treatment with the Ca^{2+} chelator BAPTA-AM inhibits astrogliosis *in vitro* (Pappalardo et al. 2014b) and *in vivo* (Gao et al. 2013), consistent with an important physiological role for the robust astroglial $[Ca^{2+}]_i$ response seen after injury (**Fig. 2.7**) (Pappalardo et al. 2014b). Our work identified a Ca^{2+} signaling cascade that contributes to glial scarring in an *in vitro* mechanical injury model similar to that previously discussed (MacFarlane and Sontheimer 1998; Pappalardo et al. 2014b; Samad et al. 2012). Gao et al. (2013) showed that the increased $[Ca^{2+}]_i$ transient in astrocytes after injury activates the protein kinase JNK, which phosphorylates transcription factor c-jun to facilitate GFAP upregulation and subsequent astrogliosis.

Recent work has also highlighted the importance of the contribution of $[Na^+]_i$ fluctuations to glial function and homeostasis, with a prominent mechanism involving the linkage of transmembrane movements of Na^+ and Ca^{2+} (Kettenmann et al. 2011; Kirischuk et al. 2012; Parpura and Verkhratsky 2012; Rose and Karus 2013; Verkhratsky et al. 2013a). Glutamate receptors and purinoceptors (Parpura and Verkhratsky 2012), as well as voltage-gated sodium channels, are known to play a role in glial Na^+ influx, and a role for sodium channels as a driver of reverse (Ca^{2+}-importing) Na^+/Ca^{2+} exchange, which has been observed in multiple glial cell types including microglia (Ifuku et al. 2007;

Kettenmann et al. 2011; Noda et al. 2013), astrocytes (Kirischuk et al. 1997; Paluzzi et al. 2007; Pappalardo et al. 2014b), and $NG2^+$ cells (Tong et al. 2009), is beginning to emerge as a common theme.

The Na^+/Ca^{2+} exchanger (NCX) operates in forward mode, transporting Na^+ ions down their concentration gradient into cells and exporting Ca^{2+} in return or, if the Na^+ electrochemical gradient is decreased or the cell is depolarized, operates in reverse mode by exporting Na^+ ions in exchange for Ca^{2+} (Annunziato et al. 2004). Thus, sodium channel activity has the capability to increase $[Ca^{2+}]_i$ via the reverse mode of NCX. Because the reversal potential of NCX in astrocytes is set at levels close to the resting membrane potential (Kirischuk et al. 1997; Reyes et al. 2012), it is possible that even small $[Na^+]_i$ increases or depolarization can rapidly trigger reverse mode of NCX operation (Kirischuk et al. 2012; Paluzzi et al. 2007), increasing $[Ca^{2+}]_i$ levels. Indeed, mechanical strain injury increases intracellular sodium, leading to NCX operating in reverse mode in cortical astrocytes (Floyd et al. 2005). As previously mentioned, sodium channel blockade attenuates astrogliosis *in vitro*, which is interestingly also reduced by blockade of the reverse (Ca^{2+}-importing) mode of NCX. A KB-R7943 concentration of 0.5 µM selectively affects the reverse mode of NCX $[IC_{50} = 1.1- 3.4$ µmol/L for reverse mode and $IC_{50} > 30$ µmol/L for forward mode] (Iwamoto et al. 1996; Persson et al. 2013a; Persson et al. 2013b); Pappalardo et al. (2014b) detailed an attenuation of injury-induced gliosis (Fig. 2.2), affecting both astroglial proliferation and migration after treatment with 0.5 µM KB-R7943. Of note, blockade of reverse Na^+/Ca^{2+} exchange decreased wound closure to a similar extent as both 10 µM TTX or Nav1.5 siRNA knockdown and there was no additional attenuation of gliosis with the combination of KB-R7943 + TTX, indicating possible non-additivity in the underlying mechanisms involved (Pappalardo et al. 2014b). Furthermore, blockade of reverse NCX activity with KB-R7943 diminished the $[Ca^{2+}]_i$ transient observed after injury to a similar extent as both TTX and Nav1.5 siRNA (**Fig. 2.6, 2.7**) (Pappalardo et al. 2014b). Thus, Na^+ flux through voltage-gated sodium channels, triggered by mechanical injury, elicits reverse operation of the Na^+/Ca^{2+} exchanger, affecting cellular motility, facilitating astrogliosis *in vitro* (**Fig. 5.1**).

A similar mechanism seems to exist in $NG2^+$ cells. Tong et al. (2009) demonstrated increased intracellular Na^+ and Ca^{2+} levels, membrane depolarizations, and enhanced migratory capacity after GABA application. Blockade or knockdown of sodium channels by siRNA significantly decreased the rise in both $[Na^+]_i$ and $[Ca^{2+}]_i$ and attenuated cell migration, and siRNA knockdown of NCX or blockade of reverse Na^+/Ca^{2+} exchange with KB-R7943 similarly decreased $[Ca^{2+}]_i$ and reduced cell migration (Tong et al. 2009).

Microglia also express NCX (Kettenmann et al. 2011) and it is possible that the functional contribution of sodium channels to effector functions (e.g. migration, phagocytosis) involves the close linkage between glial Na^+ and Ca^{2+} homeostasis. Indeed, as previously mentioned, Nav1.6 blockade (with TTX) or knockout (in *med* mice) decreases the formation of lamellipodia in ATP-activated microglia (**Fig. 1.4B**), which is the initial step in migration (Persson et al. 2014).

Sodium channel blockade additionally enhances recovery of the microglial $[Ca^{2+}]_i$ response following ATP stimulation (**Fig. 1.5C**) and decreases levels of active Rac1 (**Fig. 1.5A**) and phosphorylated MAP kinase ERK1/2 (**Fig. 1.5B**) (Persson et al. 2014). Given that both Rac1 and MAP kinase activity are modulated by levels of intracellular Ca^{2+} (Aspenstrom 2004; Chuderland et al. 2008; Price et al. 2003; Wiegert and Bading 2011), it is plausible that sodium channel blockade decreases $[Ca^{2+}]_i$ levels, resulting in attenuation of active Rac1 and phosphorylated ERK1/2 levels, subsequently inhibiting microglial migration. Thus, while the underlying mechanisms linking sodium channel activity to effector functions in glia are still incompletely understood, increasing evidence points to a link between Na^+ and Ca^{2+} signaling, with implications for the activity of the Na^+/Ca^{2+} exchanger.

5.3   THERAPEUTIC IMPLICATIONS

There is a large body of evidence detailing the favorable effect of sodium

channel blockade in animal models of neurological diseases including EAE; the

partial blockade of voltage-gated sodium channels has indeed been proposed as

a treatment strategy for MS (Waxman 2008). Previous EAE studies have shown

improved clinical status and reduction of axonal loss following treatment with a

variety of voltage-gated sodium channel blockers including phenytoin (Black et

al. 2007; Craner et al. 2005; Lo et al. 2002; Lo et al. 2003), lamotrigine (Bechtold

et al. 2006), carbamazepine (Black et al. 2007), safinamide (Morsali et al. 2013),

and flecainide (Bechtold et al. 2004; Bechtold et al. 2005; Morsali et al. 2013).

Additionally, phenytoin protects spinal cord axons, reduces gray and white matter

destruction surrounding the lesion, and improves functional recovery after

contusion-induced SCI (Hains et al. 2004) and phenytoin, riluzole, and mexilitine

have all shown to improve outcomes in murine models of SCI, with decreased

free radicals and spinal cord edema, and improved locomotion (Ates et al. 2007).

It has been proposed that inhibition of sodium channel activity by state-

dependent sodium channel-blocking agents is neuroprotective by two or more

different mechanisms: firstly, by directly blocking the persistent sodium influx in

neurons, which can drive reverse Na^+/Ca^{2+} exchange, leading to irreversible

axonal damage due to high $[Ca^{2+}]_i$ levels (Bechtold and Smith 2005; Stys et al.

1992), and second, by modulating the response of immune cells and/or glial cells

to neuroinflammation via sodium channel blockade. Aside from glia, immune

cells such as macrophages (Black et al. 2013; Carrithers et al. 2011; Carrithers et al. 2009; Carrithers et al. 2007; Craner et al. 2005; Schmidtmayer et al. 1994),

and lymphocytes (DeCoursey et al. 1985; Decoursey et al. 1987; Fraser et al.

2008; Lai et al. 2000; Lo et al. 2012) also express sodium channels. That the

observed effects of sodium channel blockade is in part attributable to

noncanonical sodium channel functioning is consistent with the observations that

flecainide (Bechtold et al. 2004; Morsali et al. 2013), safinamide (Morsali et al.

2013), phenytoin (Black et al. 2007; Craner et al. 2005), and carbamazepine

(Black et al. 2007) reduce levels of reactive microglia in EAE. Given that a robust

increase in Nav1.6 occurs in activated microglia and macrophages in both EAE

and MS and is related to phagocytic and migratory activity and

chemokine/cytokine release (Black et al. 2009; Black and Waxman 2012; Craner

et al. 2005; Persson et al. 2014), it is plausible that the protective effect of

sodium channel-blocking agents in neuroinflammation is in part attributable to the

functional role of sodium channels in reactive microglia. The possible effects of

astrocytic sodium channel blockade in CNS disease in vivo have been less

studied until the present work, though immunomodulatory roles for astrocytes in

the injured CNS are well-recognized (Brosnan and Raine 2013; Dong and

Benveniste 2001; Nair et al. 2008; Okun et al. 2009; Sofroniew 2014; Sofroniew

2015a).

Based on the preclinical rodent studies in EAE, there have been two

clinical trials in the U.K. examining the neuroprotective effects of sodium channel

blockade. In an early trial, the anticonvulsant state-dependent sodium channel

blocking agent lamotrigine was tested for efficacy in neuroprotection in the first clinical trial of this type, in patients with secondary progressive MS (Kapoor et al. 2010). One hundred and twenty patients (87 female, 33 male) were treated for 2 years with lamotrigine (target dose 400 mg/day) or placebo. The mean age was 50 years, with a mean disease duration of around 20 years, and median expanded disability status scale (EDSS) of 6.0. Neuroprotection is assumed to slow down tissue loss in the CNS (Barkhof and Filippi 2009; Fazekas et al. 2007); thus, the rate of change of cerebral volume was chosen as the primary trial outcome. Interpretation of the findings is complicated, but the group treated with lamotrigine performed significantly better in an ambulatory test (25-foot timed walk) in comparison with the control group. These positive findings occurred despite a reduction in brain volume and there was no efficacy in the other 5 clinical outcomes measured. The effect on brain volume was not anticipated at trial design, thus it confounded the primary outcome measure based on protection from loss of brain volume. However, a reduction in swelling would be expected based on the anti-inflammatory effects of sodium channel blockade and the demonstration of 'pronounced inflammation' in the brain during secondary progressive MS (Frischer et al. 2009), which could contribute to changes in brain volume. Balanced against these findings is the observation that lamotrigine therapy was less well tolerated by patients than predicted, and only 48% of patients in the treated group took the drug throughout the trial due to a perceived worsening of function. Patients with a higher EDSS score at baseline were especially susceptible to treatment related side effects, as they tolerated only lower lamotrigine concentrations. This worsening may be attributable to the suppressive effects of sodium channel blockade on neuronal activity (Kapoor et al. 2010)

Recently, the results of a second phase 2 clinical study investigating the potentially neuroprotective effects of sodium channel blockade with the antiepileptic drug phenytoin in acute optic neuritis were released (Raftopoulos et al. 2016). This study randomly assigned 86 patients (63 female, 23 male) with acute optic neuritis, within 14 days of onset of visual loss, to phenytoin or placebo. The principal study finding was that the reduction in mean retinal nerve fiber layer (RNFL) thickness was about 30% lower at 6 months in eyes affected with acute optic neuritis relative in the phenytoin group compared with the placebo group. The study was interpreted as supporting neuroprotection, although a number of factors (e.g. absence of earlier outcome measurement, small sample size) underscore the need for cautious interpretation of the results (Saidha and Calabresi 2016).

Although the clinical trials examining the neuroprotective effects of sodium channel blockers thus far have yielded less robust results than perhaps expected, there was some evidence of efficacy, and combined with preclinical rodent studies, it is still reasonable to expect that sodium channel blockade may have positive therapeutic potential in MS. It is therefore important to address the obvious discrepancy between these previous findings and our *in vivo* work (**Chapter 4**): lack of sodium channel Nav1.5 in astrocytes leads to significantly worsened clinical outcomes and increased inflammation in EAE. There are several factors to consider: firstly, this worsened effect was only observed in female mice. Male mice lacking astrocytic Nav1.5 did not fare significantly worse than male WT mice. Importantly, it appears that all previous studies demonstrating a favorable effect of sodium channel blockade in EAE were performed using male rodents (Bechtold et al. 2004; Bechtold et al. 2006; Black et al. 2007; Craner et al. 2005; Lo et al. 2002; Lo et al. 2003; Morsali et al. 2013). It is possible that EAE studies including both male and female animals would yield less favorable effects of nonselective sodium channel blockers. Consistent with this, a recent study examining the effects of selective sodium channel blockade (Nav1.2, Nav1.4, Nav1.6) in female mice found worsened clinical outcomes in EAE (Stevens et al. 2013). Whether the less positive than expected results in human clinical trials (majority female patients) are due to astrocyte sodium channel functioning is not clear. It seems likely that sodium channels play cell-specific roles, conferring both beneficial and detrimental effects to the outcomes in neurological disease. It is also possible, though speculative currently, that sodium channel blockade has differing therapeutic benefit in a sex-dependent manner. Thus, isotype-selective sodium channel blockade might by the best method to achieve maximum therapeutic potential in neuroinflammation. With this focus on developing sodium channel isotype-specific blockers, it is increasingly relevant to assess the roles of individual sodium channel isoforms in glia (e.g. Nav1.6 in microglia, Nav1.5 in astrocytes) and other involved cell types.

5.4   SUGGESTED FURTHER RESEARCH

There are numerous studies that would expand upon the results described here and further the knowledge regarding the mechanisms underlying the functional roles of sodium channels in glia. It is important to determine whether the sexual dimorphism seen in EAE with astrocyte Nav1.5 knockout mice is attributable to a functional role of Nav1.5 in modulating the neuroprotective effects of estrogen, due to inherent sex-specific cellular properties, or a combination of both. Given that ERα signaling in astrocytes modulates estrogen-mediated neuroprotection at least in part by affecting astrocyte cytokine and chemokine production (Spence et al. 2013), it would be relevant to perform *in vitro* neuroinflammatory assays (using e.g. TNFα stimulation) in the presence and absence of estrogen and TTX/Nav1.5 siRNA to determine whether sodium channels mediate release of inflammatory mediators (CCL2, CCL7, many others) in astrocytes. It would also be useful to perform further histological examination of astrocyte Nav1.5 KO mice with EAE to determine if there are changes in chemokine/cytokine production (e.g. CCL2), estrogen signaling (e.g. ERα), or BBB permeability (e.g. AQP4) compared to WT mice with EAE.

To determine whether gonadal hormones play a role in the different sex effects observed, an EAE experiment could be performed in which estrogen or placebo treatment is administered to male astrocyte Nav1.5 KO mice and male WT mice. It would be expected (and has been previously shown) that estrogen treatment would provide protection to WT male mice in EAE. However, if Nav1.5 in astrocytes is partly responsible for mediating this neuroprotective effect, there would be little difference between estrogen- and placebo-treated mice lacking astrocytic Nav1.5. Preliminary data shows that there may be merit to this study (**Fig. 5.2A, B**), and further investigation is warranted. It would also be relevant to determine if Nav1.5 plays a sex-specific role due to differing properties inherent to either male or female astrocytes. *In vitro* studies, such as those described in **Chapter 2** (which used astrocytes mixed from both male and female rats), could be performed using separate astrocytes from male or female animals to determine whether the functional role of Nav1.5 in astrocytes varies depending on sex-specific cellular properties, rather than external hormonal influences. Additionally, male versus female astrocytes could be exposed to estrogens early in development to investigate whether this triggers a persistent functional difference in the role of Nav1.5 in astrocytes, irrespective of sex of origin.

While all the data presented here are consistent with a role of Nav1.5 in shaping the response of astrocytes to injury and disease, it is important to investigate the reason our *in vivo* and *in vitro* data show seemingly divergent functional outcomes regarding the role of Nav1.5 in astrogliosis. We show that Nav1.5 plays an important role in an *in vitro* model of glial injury by triggering reverse mode operation of the Na^+-Ca^{2+} exchanger (NCX), leading to fluctuations in $[Ca^{2+}]_i$, likely affecting downstream astrocyte functions such as process extension and proliferation, which contribute to wound closure (**Chapter 2**). Conversely, in EAE, lack of Nav1.5 in astrocytes resulted in increased astroglial response (i.e. increased GFAP expression), increased inflammation, and markedly worsened clinical outcomes (**Chapter 4**). As previously discussed in

Chapter 4, the two studies use different methods to stimulate astrogliosis – one

using an *in vitro* model of traumatic injury and the other a model of *in vivo* CNS

neuroinflammatory disease. It may be useful to produce an *in vitro* model more

consistent with inflammation, perhaps by adding inflammatory mediators (e.g.

TNFα, LPS) and/or other immune cells, such as microglia, to determine if this

environment produces a different outcome regarding the role of astrocytic Nav1.5

in the wound healing experiment and other assays described in Chapter 2.

Another consideration is that astrocytes were physically injured in the *in vitro*

scratch assay, while they presumably remain intact during EAE. It could be

worthwhile to perform an *in vitro* experiment in which cells remain uninjured, such

as a transwell migration assay with a chemoattractant, in the presence and

absence of TTX/Nav1.5 siRNA to determine if Nav1.5 plays a similar role in

injured versus uninjured astrocytes *in vitro*. Finally, it would be interesting to

employ a more traumatic model of neurological disease, such as SCI, to further

investigate the functional outcomes of astrocyte Nav1.5 KO *in vivo*. Previous SCI

studies have shown favorable effects on lesion size, functional outcomes, and

axonal loss with sodium channel blockade, though as in previous EAE studies,

only male animals were used (Ates et al. 2007; Hains et al. 2004). It is plausible

that Nav1.5 plays a differing role in the function of reactive astrocytes depending

on type and severity of disease or injury, as astrogliosis itself is a heterogeneous,

highly context-dependent process.

Given the central role of glia in CNS health and disease, there is a need

for further understanding of the physiologically relevant roles of glial sodium

channels and characterization of molecular pathways governing the functional

roles of sodium channels in these cells. There has been much work performed in

cell culture, but further *in vivo* studies are of crucial importance for determination

of the therapeutic implications of targeting glial sodium channels in neurological

disorders such as MS.

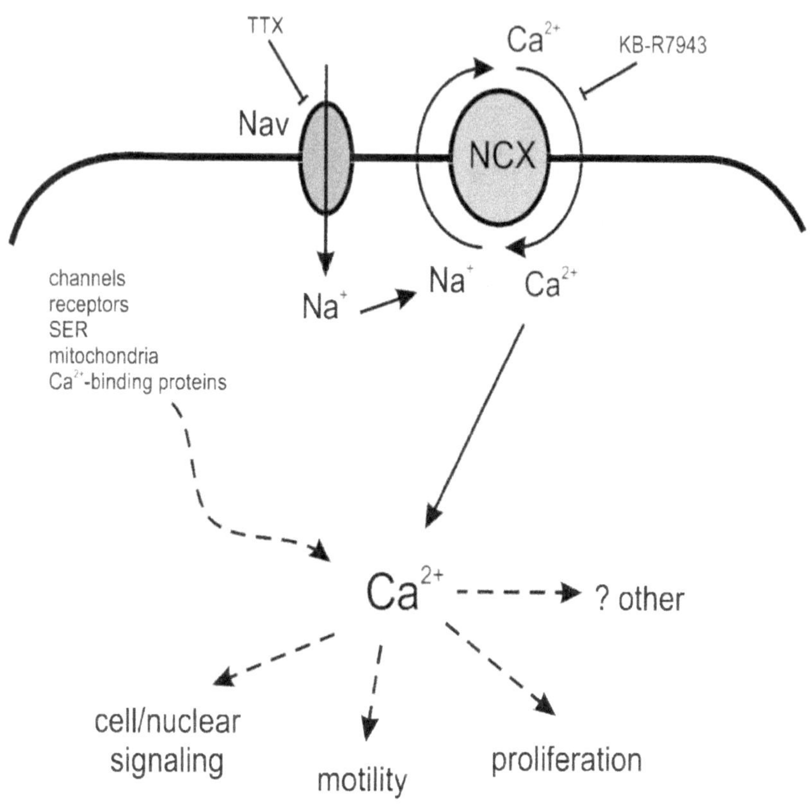

Figure 5.1. Schematic of putative pathway of sodium channel contribution to intracellular Ca^{2+} levels and downstream pathways. Depolarization of glial membrane leads to activation of voltage-gated sodium channels (Nav) allowing influx of Na$^+$. Increased [Na$^+$]$_i$ induces reverse operation of the sodium-calcium exchanger (NCX), contributing to the level of [Ca^{2+}]$_i$. Ca^{2+} signaling initiates downstream effects on cellular functions. Blockade of sodium channels with tetrodotoxin (TTX) and reverse operation of NCX with KB-R7943 attenuates [Ca^{2+}]$_i$ levels. [Modified from Persson et al. (2014) and Pappalardo et al. (2016)].

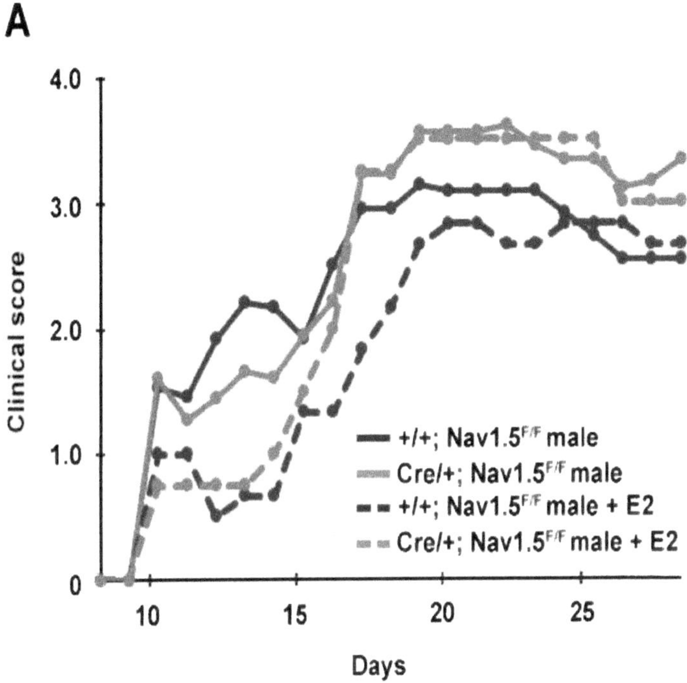
A
Clinical score
4.0
3.0
2.0
1.0
0
+/+; Nav1.5$^{F/F}$ male
Cre/+; Nav1.5$^{F/F}$ male
+/+; Nav1.5$^{F/F}$ male + E2
Cre/+; Nav1.5$^{F/F}$ male + E2
10
15
20
25
Days

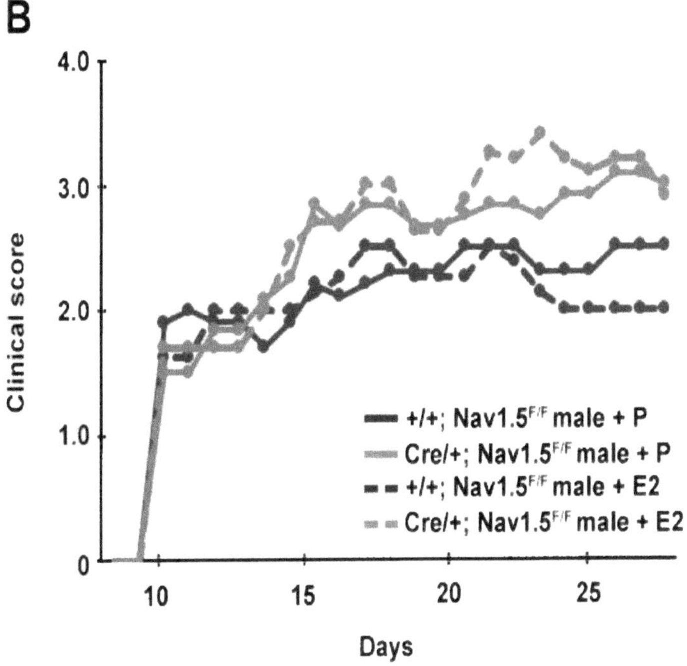
B
Clinical score
4.0
3.0
2.0
1.0
0
+/+; Nav1.5$^{F/F}$ male + P
Cre/+; Nav1.5$^{F/F}$ male + P
+/+; Nav1.5$^{F/F}$ male + E2
Cre/+; Nav1.5$^{F/F}$ male + E2
10
15
20
25
Days

Figure 5.2 – Preliminary observations examining the effect of estrogen therapy on clinical course of male Nav1.5 astrocyte knockout and control mice. (A) While both estrogen-treated male control mice (+/+; Nav1.5$^{F/F}$; dashed purple line) and estrogen-treated male astrocyte Nav1.5 knockout mice (Cre/+: Nav1.5$^{F/F}$; dashed orange line) exhibit delayed EAE onset compared to untreated male control mice (+/+; Nav1.5$^{F/F}$; purple line) and untreated male astrocyte Nav1.5 knockout mice (Cre/+: Nav1.5$^{F/F}$; orange line), estrogen-treated male KO mice lose any protective effect around day 15 and have no distinguishable difference in disease severity compared to untreated male KO mice. In contrast, estrogen-treated male WT mice exhibit a prolonged rescue from disease compared to untreated male WT mice. Data represent n=4 animals for each of the four groups. Estrogen pellets were inserted at day 7, prior to EAE onset. **(B)** Estrogen-treated male astrocyte Nav1.5 knockout mice (Cre/+: Nav1.5$^{F/F}$; dashed orange line) display no protective effect in EAE compared to placebo-treated male astrocyte Nav1.5 knockout mice (Cre/+: Nav1.5$^{F/F}$; orange line). In contrast, estrogen-treated male WT mice (+/+; Nav1.5$^{F/F}$; dashed purple line) display some protection from disease (beginning day 23) compared to placebo-treated male WT mice (+/+; Nav1.5$^{F/F}$; purple line). Data represent n=6 animals for each of the four groups. Estrogen and placebo pellets were inserted at day 17, after EAE onset.